CW00568345

AYURVEDA FOR LIFE

AYURVEDA FOR LIFE

A BEGINNER'S GUIDE TO BALANCE AND VITALITY

Monica Bloom

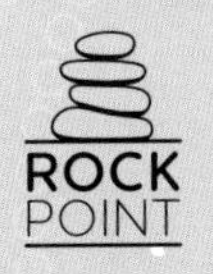

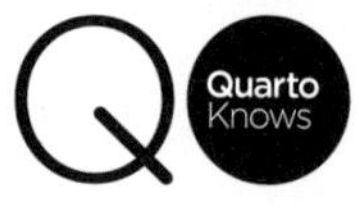

First published in 2021 by Rock Point,
an imprint of The Quarto Group,
142 West 36th Street, 4th Floor,
New York, NY 10018, USA
T (212) 779-4972 F (212) 779-6058
www.QuartoKnows.com

Rock Point titles are also available at discount for retail, wholesale, promotional, and bulk purchase. For details, contact the Special Sales Manager by email at specialsales@quarto.com or by mail at The Quarto Group, Attn: Special Sales Manager, 100 Cummings Center Suite 265D, Beverly, MA 01915, USA.

Library of Congress Cataloging-in-Publication Data

Names: Bloom, Monica, author.
Title: Ayurveda for life : a beginner's guide to balance and vitality / Monica Bloom.
Description: New York : Rock Point, 2021. | Series: Live well | Summary: "In Ayurveda for Life, learn how to integrate the original self-care practice into your busy life, by aligning your body, mind, and spirit"—Provided by publisher.
Identifiers: LCCN 2021004609 (print) | LCCN 2021004610 (ebook) | ISBN 9781631067266 (hardcover) | ISBN 9780760368763 (ebook)
Subjects: LCSH: Medicine, Ayurvedic—Popular works. | Mind and body therapies. | Self-care, Health—Popular works.
Classification: LCC R605 .B62 2021 (print) | LCC R605 (ebook) | DDC 615.5/38—dc23
LC record available at https://lccn.loc.gov/2021004609
LC ebook record available at https://lccn.loc.gov/2021004610

10 9 8 7 6 5 4 3 2 1

ISBN: 978-1-63106-726-6

Publisher: Rage Kindelsperger
Creative Director: Laura Drew
Managing Editor: Cara Donaldson
Editor: Keyla Pizarro-Hernández
Cover and Interior Design: Lauren Vajda

Printed in China

DEDICATED TO ALELLA

Share your big dreams, Lovely.
Awesome people in life will show up
and help you make them come true.

Contents

Introduction

Life meets work. Work meets life. You play many different roles in a day, but you are the same person who transitions through all of them. You are the central hub of your life and when your mind, body, and spirit work better, everything around you will work better.

So, you picked up this book for a reason. Maybe you're curious about what the heck Ayurveda is, but I sense you're here because you want to do better in your life somehow. You want more daily joy. You want to feel healthy in your body. You want to feel like you're bigger than your stresses. You want to feel in control of yourself. You want to be a happy person for your spouse and kids. You're ready to create a better version of yourself.

Good! Then you're in the right place. This book is to educate and inspire you to *create a vibrant life on your terms*. May it ignite joy, surprise, and delight while giving you direction to help you feel good each day in your mind, body, and spirit.

HOW TO USE THIS BOOK

The book has three parts: Roots, Rise, and Bloom.

Roots give you the foundation. The roots are the building blocks, so you are supported with the right knowledge. When you have the knowledge, you have it forever, which gives you empowerment to make choices for your own health and life.

Rise is your growth. Once you have strong roots, you can grow! This is where you apply actions to help you change and evolve. Grow from the roots of your new knowledge and sprout above the surface, stretching higher and higher.

Bloom will help you flourish. Once you have strong roots, and the tools to rise, you're ready to bloom! You'll bloom with advanced practices and additional perspectives to help you thrive.

Accessible, daily Ayurveda is what we are going to focus on because that's where you have the most empowerment to change your life. This book is a blend of my Ayurvedic knowledge and what I've learned from having to wrangle a busy lifestyle and make it work for me. I hope what I've experienced and learned on my journey will help make your journey easier and full of joy as you go.

There are insights and "Bring It to Life" exercises throughout the book to help you practice Ayurveda techniques in your daily life, so my suggestion is to use this book like a life manual. Make it yours. Write in the margins, highlight it, or slap a sticky note on anything that inspires you or resonates with you. Love it up.

If you want to zip through and do some of the practices right away, you can, but you'll do better with some context. I suggest you begin with the roots. When you have strong Ayurvedic roots, you'll be so much more empowered because you'll have the knowledge—forever.

A LITTLE ABOUT ME

In writing, teaching, and practicing Ayurveda for over a decade, I have found that the most impactful Ayurveda is simple and daily. Much like you, I'm a worker bee, juggling several things at once and striving to be the best version of myself. My superpower is teaching people how to use Ayurveda to manage a busy lifestyle and find balance in the workplace. I live at the intersection of where Ayurveda meets the daily grind.

I see Ayurveda from the eyes of a mom (human and fur babies), wife, corporate business leader, and small business owner in a highly competitive environment and fast-paced lifestyle. I ended up burning out over the years. But by practicing Ayurveda, I've learned how to strike a balance to take care of myself, be there for my family, teach my team, grow business(es), and spend time on things that matter most to me.

I also believe in energy work, spirituality, and a power beyond what we experience with our senses. I personally balance the daily tangible practices with the more spiritual. I love my abundance of crystals, I chant with my mala beads, I light powder on fire, I talk to the universe and my higher self, I place "wealth" symbols in my house and get busted by my husband, I diffuse essential oils, and I have a Vedic astrology advisor (thanks, Joey! *rock on*).

I love all that stuff, but you won't find much of that in this book because these mystical things were not the things that changed my life first!

To make big shifts, I had to change my diet, my mind-set, my actions, my schedule, and my energy, and, most of all, I had to make myself a priority. Because without those basic changes, I could not be of service to anyone else.

To start, let's get your daily stuff together, establish your roots, help you rise, and nourish your blooms so that you can stretch up and reach the stars.

So, my friend, get ready to embark on a journey that goes inside yourself and then radiates outward to all you do and all you love.

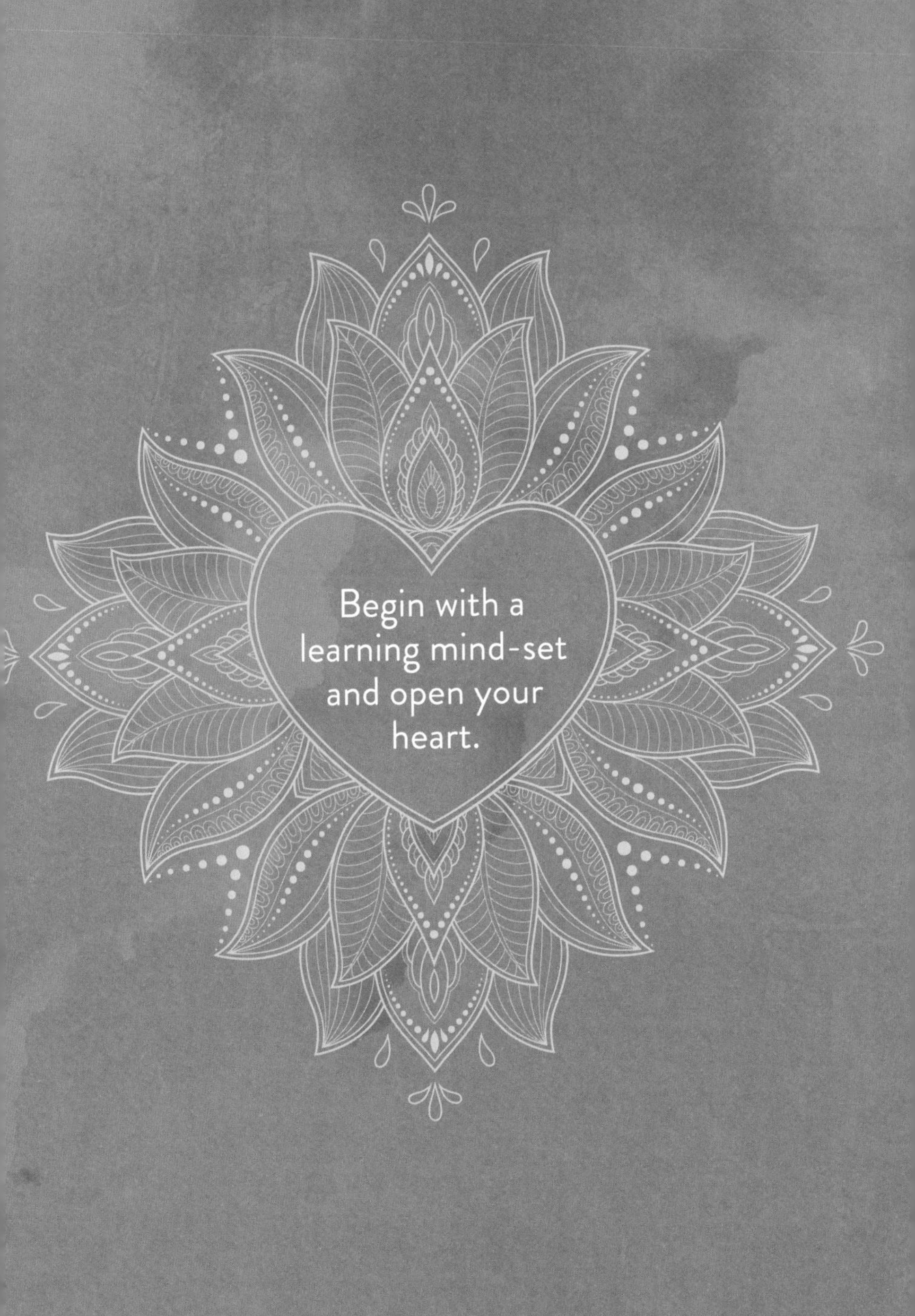
Begin with a
learning mind-set
and open your
heart.

Part 1

ROOTS

CHAPTER 1

Establish Your Roots

Let's establish several roots to get you started! These roots are unshakable. These are the things you will look back to often in life to bring you back to center, back to balance, back to your full strength. Life can be unpredictable at times. There will be moments when you feel "uprooted," when internal or external changes make you feel like you are on "shaky ground." It's just part of life. All things are always in flux and in a state of change, but when you realize that you can come back to your roots at any time, it gives you the security you need to keep growing, rising, and blooming—as you move forward to create your best self.

So, right off the bat as one of your roots, take whatever you already think you know about diet, lifestyle, and self-care, and put it aside.

Be open to a brand-new way to do life. Many of these concepts will be different than anything you've ever heard before. But that's good, because you didn't pick up an Ayurveda book to be told the same old things. You picked up this book so you could have empowerment to create a better life and better health, so in order to do that, you need a mind-set shift. Ready? Here we go.

Many of us have been taught black-and-white thinking—right or wrong, good or bad, on or off, this or that. We tend to want to follow these rules to fall into the right bucket or to execute one specific thing perfectly to get a desired result. But black-and-white thinking is so limiting! It creates a way of thinking that makes us feel like we only have two options. And if we don't like one of those two options, then what's left?

The gray area.

Who wants to be in the gray area?! Nobody. Everybody runs screaming from the gray area. The gray area is no-man's-land and it can feel unsettling not to know our next move. The gray area of thinking can make us feel like an indecisive loser.

Years ago, in the midst of my own healing journey, I found myself in the gray area all the time! I was often so uncomfortable with myself. Eventually, I got so sick of feeling like an indecisive loser, so I changed my mind-set.

I told myself a new story so that instead of feeling stressed, my new story made me feel expansive and positive. A little change in perspective, a little mind-set shift, went a long way for me and it will go a long way for you, too!

Embrace a rainbow mind-set. Oh! *your soul lights up* Rainbow space is where all possibilities exist!

So, my friend, from now on, the space between black and white is not gray, it's rainbow. Rainbow is the mind-set where you can create options. You know there are better ways. You know you are unlimited. And you know you don't know everything.

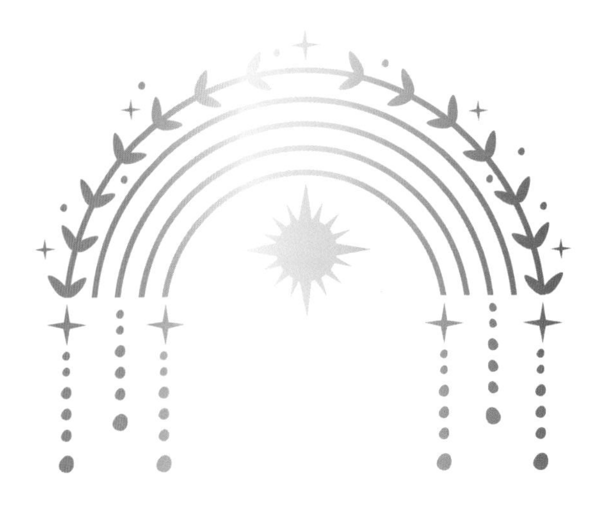

I decided to choose a more positive outlook and renamed this unknown gray area the "rainbow space."

Rainbow mind-set is where you explore options that you didn't even know existed! If you don't like the two black and white options, invent a third, a fourth, or a fifth. With a rainbow mind-set, you no longer have three choices: black, white, or heck-no gray. You have infinite options out there for you! When you realize most of life is rainbow space (not black and white!), your lens becomes more expansive, more colored, and so does your life. As you begin this new journey, turn on your rainbow mind-set.

Activate rainbow mind-set by being flexible. Be open. Be a creator. Be ready to try new things.

Say yes to an unknown path that could lead somewhere awesome—if it doesn't, you can always turn around. That is rainbow. Use your rainbow mind-set to be ready to learn something new, and explore what is unknown to you, with trust and optimism.

Here's an example of using rainbow mind-set: In Ayurveda, calories don't exist. That's right, Ayurveda does not have calories (see page 76). Instead of measuring food and counting it, we pay attention to the digestive power of the unique person. We focus on the types of food that will benefit the unique individual. We promote eating in a positive mood. We make sure to eat at the right times according to nature's clock. Ayurveda takes the numbers out of food, so you can intuitively feel what your body needs and make choices accordingly.

For many people this no-calories thing is mind-blowing and freeing. *That* is how I invite you to see your unique self, your life, and to experience this way of living. Don't try to jam yourself tight into a limited way of thinking. All possibilities are there, and in Ayurveda, everything depends. There are some basic guidelines and rules to give you structure, but much of using Ayurveda is by your own design. This is all about you.

Trust as you go that the information will unfold perfectly for where you are in this moment.

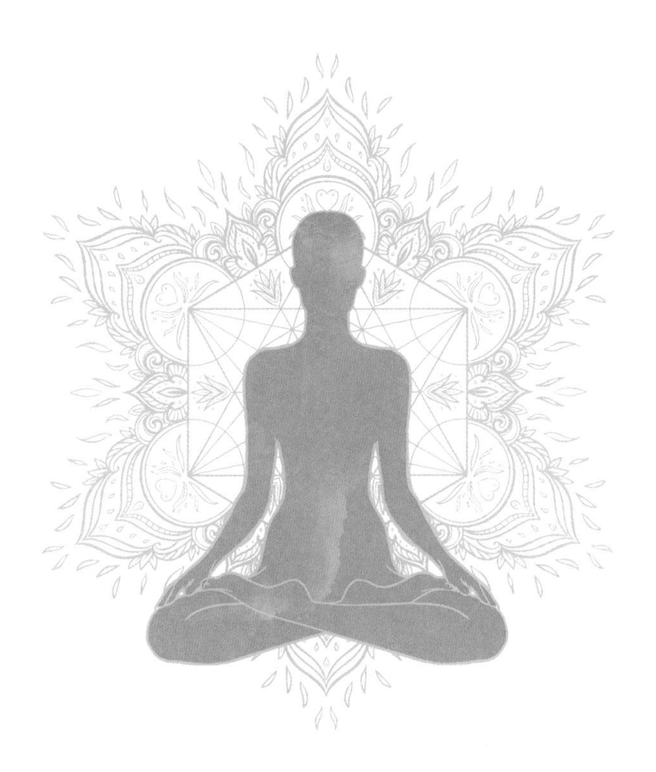

What Is Ayurveda?

Ayurveda is balancing your health according to who you are as a unique individual in mind, body, and spirit. It is the science or knowledge of life. It is the understanding of who we are becoming in this lifetime for the sake of giving our best service and contribution to the world.

Ayurveda covers everything—your food, your schedule, your emotions, your mental health, your physical health, your spiritual health, your environment, your relationships, your illnesses, and your cures. Ayurveda helps us achieve longevity through various methods, including daily self-care, diet, lifestyle guidelines, therapies, and remedies. It focuses on prevention, but it can cure disease and illness.

Ayurveda is thousands of years old and is India's original medical system. In India, people go to medical schools to study Ayurveda just like doctors do in the West. It's not a light and fluffy, New Agey thing. It is true healthcare with ancient roots and methods that have a massive impact on preventing and curing health problems.

Why is Ayurveda so passionate about our longevity, anyway? The reason we want to live a long time is so that we have time to fulfill our dharma, our purpose in this lifetime, or "the essence of our existence." Think of dharma as being of service. We are all on this planet to serve someone in some way, whether we are aware of it or not. Maybe your dharma is the business you started or the volunteer work you do or the books you write. Maybe your dharma is to be a loving, connected parent to your kids. It's different for everybody, but it's all based on service generosity and our contribution in this lifetime.

When life is devoid of dharma (or giving service), we suffer. It is said that when we are without dharma there cannot be any happiness in life. You might recognize it as feeling "soulless" or "lost." If you've ever been there and gotten yourself out of it, I am willing to bet that when you started giving and serving in some way, you started to feel better.

In a nutshell, Ayurveda teaches you how to live long enough and well enough to do your work—your life's purpose.

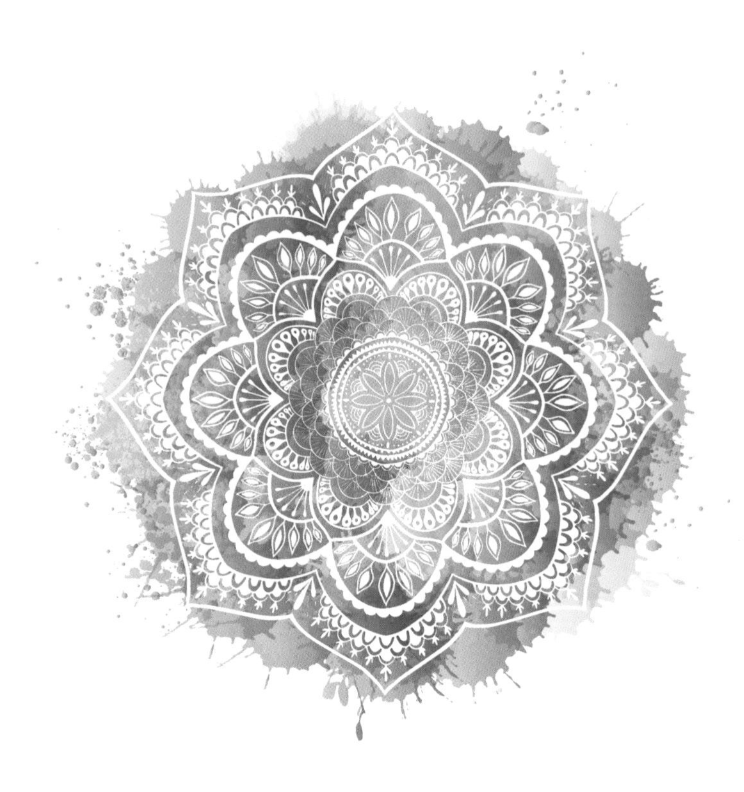

It Depends

In Ayurveda, there is no one set cure or solution for anything or anyone.

"It depends" is the quintessential phrase used in Ayurveda because everyone is so uniquely different that you can't treat them all the same way. Even if two people have the same health problem, the approach, therapies, and substances used will be different.

Everything depends, including the season, the person's digestion, daily routine, diet, mind-set, environment, past habits, and so on. All of these will determine the method, the vehicle, and the substances of healing. Because one size does not fit all, Ayurveda says, "It depends."

Sound a little complicated? Well, it is. Remember, this is a big ol' medical science! But again, you don't need to know all this to be healthy and happy. Just understand that what works for you might not work for someone else and vice versa. Ayurveda is highly personalized.

Here's a hypothetical example: You eat salad in the summer and feel fine, but in winter, you feel bloated. There's nothing wrong with salad and nothing wrong with you. But eating salad for you depends on the season. In the summer, when the weather is warm, you can digest a cooling salad because the cool balances the heat. In the winter months, both the weather and the salad are cold, which makes it tougher on digestion, which causes you to feel bloated. See? It depends. When you eat salad in summer, you feel fine; when you eat salad in winter, not fine.

I share this to make sure that if you try a new diet or exercise program that doesn't work for you, it doesn't mean there's something wrong with you. You are unique and everything depends.

Learn to honor yourself, ask better questions, and have compassion for others with the knowledge that all of life "depends." It's not black and white. **rainbow!**

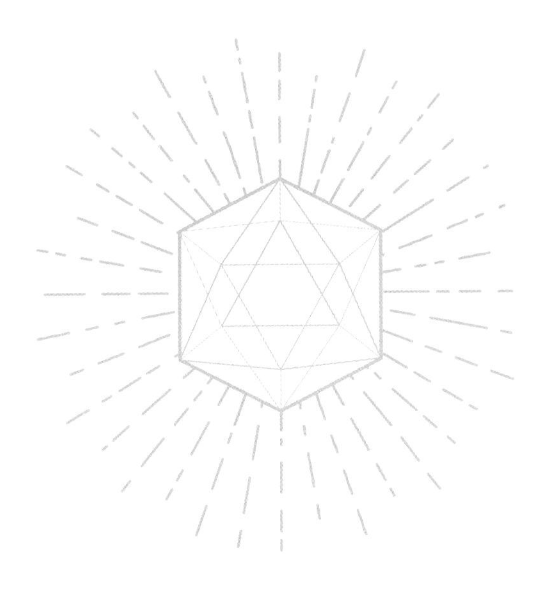

Macrocosm versus Microcosm

Ayurveda says that nature plays a crucial role in our well-being because of the macrocosm versus microcosm philosophy. This philosophy asserts that the large nature (macrocosm) is made of the same things as the small nature (microcosm). In Ayurveda, it is said that from the giant universe, down to our planet Earth, all the way down to our bodies and inside our tiny cells, only five things exist: space, air, fire, water, and earth. These are the five great elements.

So, everything all the way from the macro (universe!) down to the tiny micro (us!) is made of just those five elements. There are an indefinite amount of ways the elements combine to form everything: The sky. The oceans. The mountains. The trees. The rocks. The rain. The leaves. People. Tiny bugs. Therefore, we are closely connected to and influenced by the larger nature. When we surround ourselves with environments, substances, and foods that come directly from these five natural elements, we feel awesome!

Think about the difference between air-conditioning and having the windows open. Or the difference between a hike through a redwood forest versus a stroll through an indoor mall. Different, right?!

This is why, when we plan vacations, we tend to choose nature-filled locations and activities like national parks, lakeside cabins, ski resorts, lush surroundings, desert retreats, or beach time for the sake of experiencing the elements in their fullest. Most times, we feel happy, relaxed, and peaceful on vacation because we've taken conscious time to connect to and be in nature.

So, why don't we do that in our daily lives? Instead, we spend much of our time sitting in offices or our houses for work (jobs are good) and take care of our families (families are good), but knowing the outdoors is where we feel best and is healing for us, we can make a conscious choice to spend more time there, daily!

Because macrocosm (big nature) and microcosm (small nature, like us) are made of the same things (space, air, fire, water, earth), our bodies and minds thrive when we are "fed" natural things like the outdoors, natural foods, and natural ingredients, and when we spend time with each other. We balance out mentally, emotionally, and physically when we spend time in natural surroundings often.

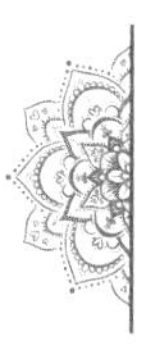

BALANCING ACT: *Intentionally get outside daily. Take a morning or an evening walk (your dog will thank you!). Or take a short break at work in the afternoon, around 2 or 3 p.m.*

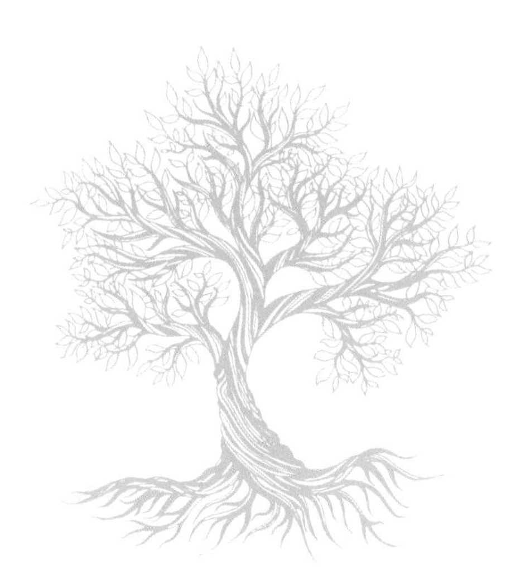

Nature and Ayurveda

The purity of nature has an intelligence and a life force that is called *prana*.

Considering prana and the macrocosm–microcosm rule, all healing modalities in Ayurveda are natural from the purest sources. Our body recognizes these natural substances, welcomes them, and digests them in a way that balances us.

It's when we take the life force out of our days that we can get imbalanced. Some examples of this include work environments that lack natural light, computer and phone screens, processed foods (far from their natural sources!), pesticides, fake sugars, chemical products for the home or skin, and so on. As soon as we introduce substances or environments that have been fake-ified in any way from the pure five elements, we remove the natural source of intelligence—so the substance, food, or environment becomes "dead" and is not properly digested.

When we spend too much time in an unnatural environment, eating unnatural foods, using unnatural products, and not using our bodies and breath in the right way, we too can feel a little "dead." Our body will often reject these things, even giving us the impression that we are "sick," when really we just need to remove that unnatural thing. If we start bringing nature back into our foods and lifestyle, we'll do much better.

So, after we unknowingly have spent years toxifying ourselves with chemically processed foods, skin creams, screen time, the daily rat race, pollution, sodas, sugars, and alcohols (I'm being dramatic, for effect), nature is the counterbalance and the healer. We find our way back to ourselves by way of pure food, breathwork, natural healing therapies, and spending time in nature.

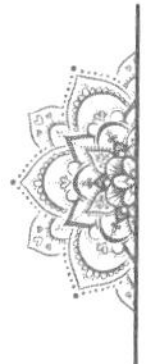

BALANCING ACT: *Find one thing that is unnatural in your diet or lifestyle that you can swap out for something that is natural. For example, choose water instead of soda, the outdoors instead of the treadmill, dates instead of candy.*

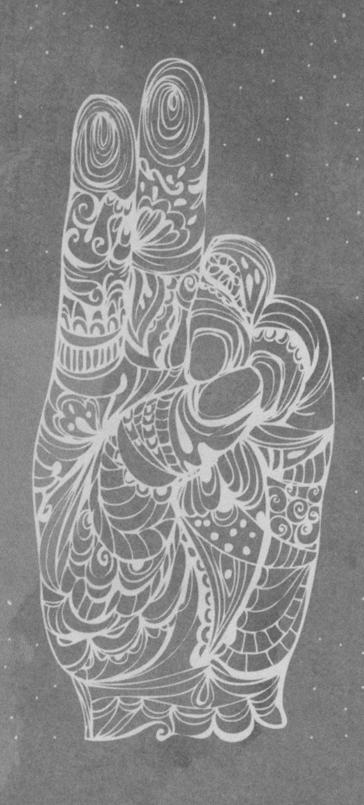

Prana is our vital life force.
We get prana from our breath, from our food, and from nature. Without sufficient prana, we feel low energy, tired, lifeless, and even depressed.

Like Increases Like

In Ayurveda, there are groupings of opposites found in nature, like hot/cold, light/heavy, and dry/wet or oily. Using these opposites, also called qualities, is how we create balance. When there is too much of the same quality, that quality increases to a level that is not good, and imbalance happens. Adding even more of the same quality will cause further imbalance.

Here's an example: When it's a cold winter day, we wouldn't intuitively jump into a cold swimming pool. Cold plus cold equals more cold and maybe hypothermia if we hang out there long enough. However, on a cold winter day, we might enjoy a warm bath or a hot tub soak, because the warm water balances the cold weather. See there? Opposites balance.

On the other hand, a hot tub, in the sun, on a 90-degree day sounds a little too hot, right? The sun, the hot water, and the outside temperature are natural elements, but the heats are all stacked up. All that heat and fire would heat you up too (macro/micro). You might get overheated and feel like you're going to pass out, you might get red in the face, or your skin might feel like it's burning. "Like increased like"—you can feel it.

The cure? Opposites! When it's hot outside, get to the cool pool. You might run (I mean walk) for your floaty and jump in—then you'd be able to handle the heat from the sun and the temperature better. In fact, it would feel amazing!

These are very obvious examples, but they illustrate how "like increases like" works. Just because something is natural, if it's not a quality (like hot/cold) that balances the person, it won't be of help and could make the situation worse.

These are great things to pay attention to in your own body. Don't doubt yourself, and trust your intuition. If you're always cold, find something to warm you up. If you feel heavy in your body, try lighter foods and body movement (both create more lightness). If you feel too light in your body, try grounding, heavy foods or slow exercise that is close to the ground (like yoga or weights). If your skin is dry, you might need more oils—on the skin and maybe in your diet, too. If you are too damp or oily (like congested, or have a lot of mucus), you need to dry out; you could do this by adding spices to your food, going to the desert, or sitting in a sauna.

See how this works? Very common things can be fixed with the "like increases like" rule. It's how Ayurveda heals, maintains good health, and prevents imbalance.

TIP: If you're not used to tapping into your body, then simply observe and start to get reacquainted with it. It will give you loads of information about what it needs.

Now that you have this root, trust what your body is telling you. Trust that you intuitively know how to care for yourself—and then follow through.

Find Balance on the Middle Path

As we strive to better our life or health, we sometimes jump to extremes to get results, such as choosing a restrictive diet or going for a big and intense exercise overhaul. An example of an extreme is completely cutting out a certain food group, like grains. Or on the flip side, only eating a certain food group, like vegetables. But, no matter how "healthy" the idea may seem, anything that is extreme is not balance. Extremes could be in quantity, quality, frequency, or duration. Extremes are not sustainable for the long term, and they do not provide balance.

Here's a silly example of an extreme: Eating a cupcake after every meal for dessert will cause some kind of imbalance—let's say weight gain. But if you ate a cupcake one time per month, would it cause the same problem? No. The problem is not the cupcake; the problem is the frequency and quantity of cupcake intake (that's fun to say, someone please start a cupcake company called "the cupcake intake"). That cupcake habit is the root cause of physical and maybe mental imbalance. We could use this cupcake example with any substance or habit.

Here are some other common examples of extremes: never working out, working out at a high intensity every day, having two glasses of wine every night, never eating warm food, eating ice cream every night, always going to bed late, always skipping lunch, or staring at a screen for ten or more hours a day. On occasion, these things will not screw you up. But if done over time, as habits, they would. Every one of them would in some way affect your physical, emotional, or mental balance. Our balance is found not on one extreme or the other, but in the middle. Think of the middle path as "the right amount."

So, my friends, walk the middle path.

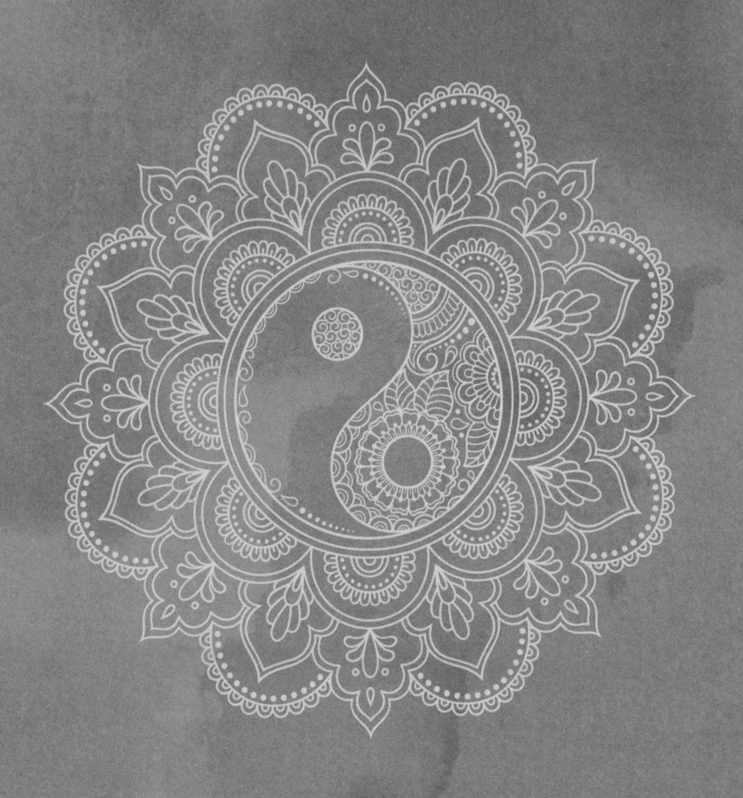

In Ayurveda, we walk the middle path. Too much or too little of anything is not good. The middle path is where we find balance.

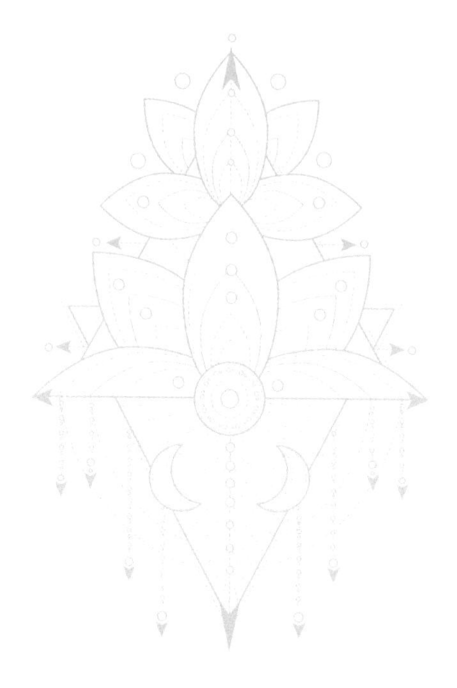

Variety and counterbalance keep the body and mind in balance. So, if you're on screens, be sure to take frequent breaks for the sake of your eyes and posture. And try not to spend the evening with your face in a screen. Work out at an intensity and duration that are sustainable for you, but not too high of an intensity that it wears down your tissues. Have sweet treats or a glass of wine sometimes—but probably not every day. Make sure your meals are well balanced with a variety of colors, flavors, and food groups.

This balance is where we find our good health and how we can achieve our best selves. Balance is not heavy on one side. Balance is even. It is the middle. Balance does not mean perfection. There is no such thing as being perfect, so chuck that expectation into the creek.

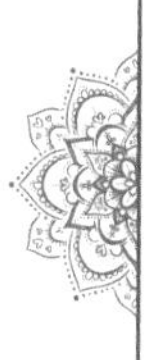

BALANCING ACT: *If anything in your life feels like an extreme, bring it back to the middle. Small changes and small wins are what you are after (not extremes) because they are sustainable, and more importantly, they create momentum and motivation to keep doing awesome things for yourself.*

BRING IT TO LIFE

- Identify one habit that feels extreme and write down how you can bring it back to the middle.
- Choose an obstacle or a challenge you are facing. Use the rainbow mind-set to come up with at least ten ways to solve the problem. Then try one of them. If it doesn't work, then you have at least nine more options to try.
- When someone asks you a question expecting a yes or no answer, reply with "it depends." And then talk to them about all possibilities.

CHAPTER 2

Hello, Self!

Oh boy! This is going to be your favorite part because you get to learn all about you! Who doesn't like to learn all about themselves? It's an instant party when you get clarity for why you are the way you are! You're just you. And you're amazing.

In a busy lifestyle, it's easy to lose our ground or confidence—or even know whether we are doing things right. This chapter will help you understand, from the roots, what makes you *you*. From this space, you can rock your natural gifts and be aware of the tendencies that hold you back.

You will no longer feel like you need to match what others are doing and instead you'll feel free to craft your own little road map of life, built uniquely for you, by you. You'll find strong roots and inner security because you'll know yourself. As a bonus, you will gain so much more appreciation, understanding, and compassion for others. Instead of them driving you bonkers, you'll see them through a different lens. This root will help us truly understand one another, as we each beat to our own drum, while at the same time honoring others and building harmonious relationships.

Let's give a little *thank you* to the differences that we each bring—like a beautiful bouquet of humans. The more different and unique, the more stunning the bouquet.

One Size Does Not Fit All

Remember the five great elements: space, air, fire, water, and earth? These five elements combine to form three energies that govern us and nature—vata, pitta, and kapha. Those three energies are called *doshas*. All five elements are in the universe, and all five elements are in the three doshas; therefore, we have all three doshas in us too.

Each one of us is a completely unique blend of the five elements.

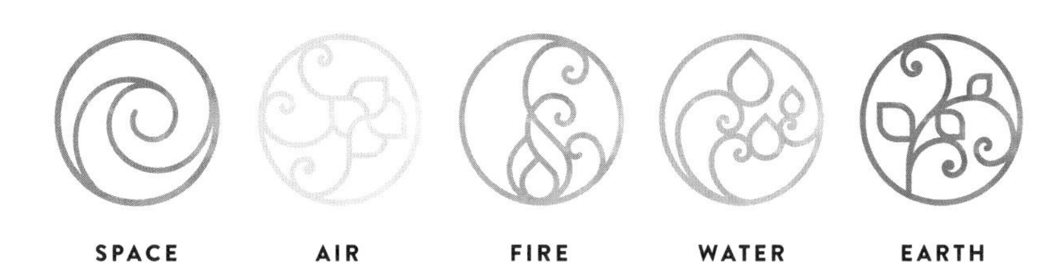

We each have our own blend of the doshas, which is why we look, act, and think differently from one another. Therefore, our body shape, tolerance for stress, perceptions, mental state, and emotions are completely unique because they are driven by which doshas are most prominent in us. It's also the reason why any particular diet, exercise regime, or remedy does not work for everyone.

Here's how three people can be different when given the same scenario. Let's say these three people are trying to put together a puzzle. Here's how each of their minds works differently:

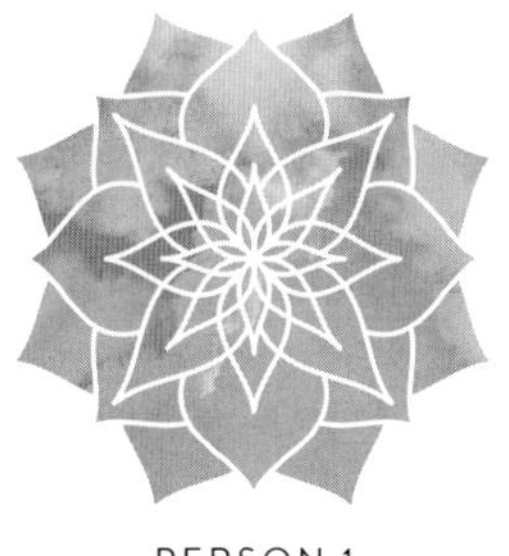

PERSON 1

PITTA

...

Creates a plan for flipping over all the pieces, organizing them by chunks of color and pattern, and finding edge pieces.

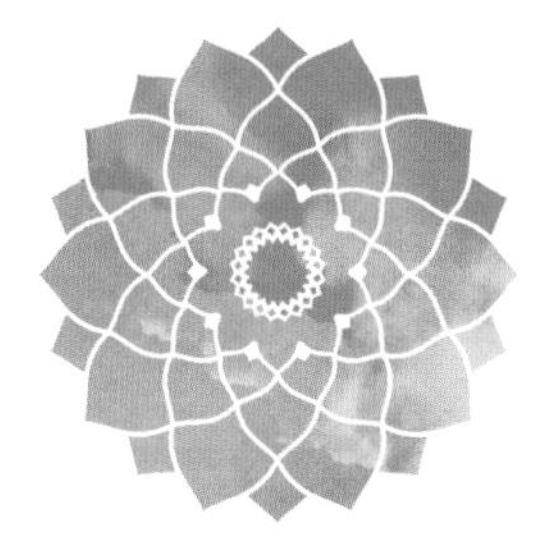

PERSON 2

KAPHA

...

Is whistling, helping flip over the pieces, and once in a while trying to get pieces to fit.

PERSON 3

VATA

...

Is already distracted and in the kitchen looking for snacks.

I'm being very stereotypical here, but can't you just see people you know in these scenarios?! Life is funny. Doshas are funny, and yet they are so rooted in truth. These examples illustrate how we are different from one another, so let's have some fun as we learn all about the doshas.

How the Doshas Shape Who You Are

As mentioned earlier, there are three doshas in us: vata, pitta, and kapha, each representing a combination of the different elements. These doshas govern our physical bodies and personalities as well as the surrounding nature. They shape precisely who you are, from your height and weight to the shape of your hands, the thickness of your hair, and the roundness and sparkliness of your eyeballs.

We have all three doshas in us, but your combination of doshas is what makes you completely unique. Living a balanced life and achieving balanced health is not created by having all three doshas in equal parts. It is about discovering your dosha(s) and keeping them balanced for your distinctive combination.

YOUR COMBINATION OF DOSHAS

Our personal combination of doshas is created at conception; it is our natural balance. If we maintain this pure balance (called *prakruti*) throughout life, it is considered optimal health. Balanced doshas means that the doshas are in the right combination for *you*.

However, the doshas are influenced by our life habits and choices, such as diet, lifestyle, schedule, the seasons, our environment, emotional traumas, and many more nuances, which can cause them to become aggravated and increase or decrease within us. The increase comes from "like increasing like," and the doshas "overflow" into areas of the body where they don't belong.

When one or more doshas increase to a level beyond what is natural for you, you feel crummy in mind or body in some way. At this stage, we would usually start seeking help for our health problems because we no longer "feel like ourselves." In fact, we *aren't* really like our natural selves anymore because the doshas have imbalanced from their natural state and are now causing

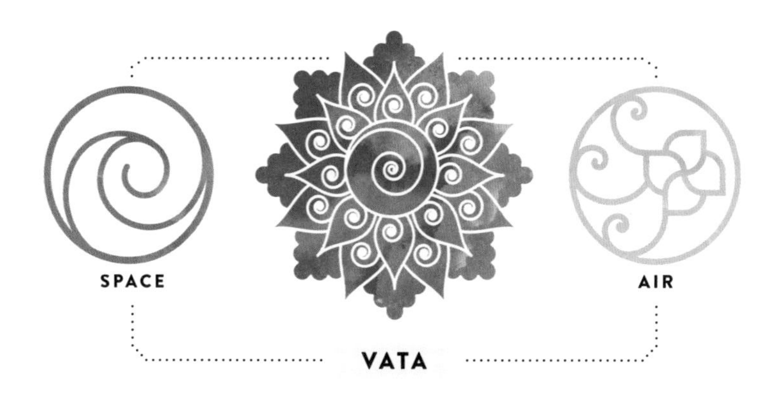
SPACE
AIR
VATA

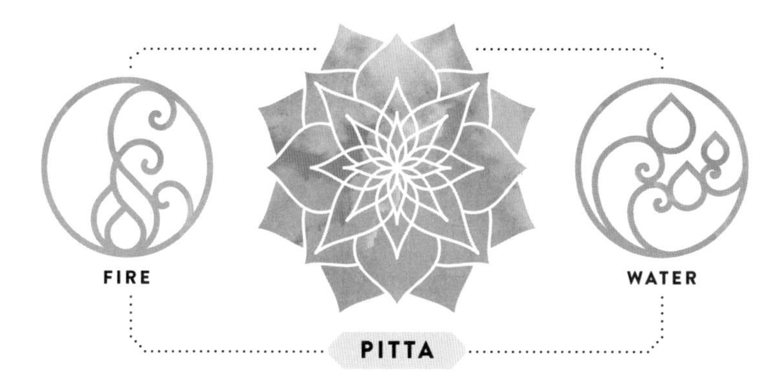
FIRE
WATER
PITTA

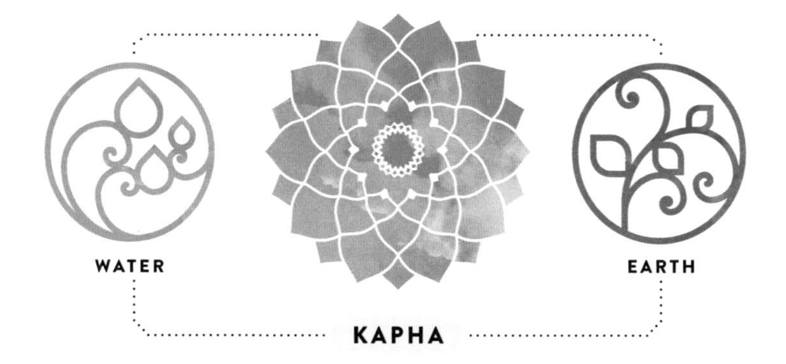
WATER
EARTH
KAPHA

problems. This is when we use "opposites to balance" and bring that dosha back into optimal balance.

The reason most of us don't have optimal health is because, over time, our external worlds and internal decisions have affected us. We acquire habits. We make choices that may or may not benefit our balance of doshas. And then, there are the things we don't know. For example, if you didn't know what a dosha was until now, how are you supposed to use the knowledge of the doshas to care for yourself? You couldn't, because you didn't know. The things that are unknown to us (Ayurveda calls it "mistaken intellect") can also be a root cause for disease or imbalance.

Prakruti, or your natural combination of doshas, stays fixed. You will always be you. You cannot turn into another dosha(s) even if you tried. It's why some people cannot gain weight no matter what. Or why naturally curly hair will always *boing* back when it gets humid or wet, despite all the straightening and flat-ironing. It's why we can't do anything about the shape of our fingers. We are fixed. Instead of critiquing or trying to change our uniqueness, let's appreciate it. Animals don't critique or compare themselves to other animals, they just thrive in their uniqueness the best they can.

The elephant does not wish it were a bird. The bird does not wish it were a lion. The lion does not try to be an elephant. They do their best with their natural physical and mental tendencies. Accept your dosha makeup. Don't spend time or energy wishing you were someone else. You are a divine combination that can never be replicated.

So don't try to put yourself in a bucket. But as you go, allow your knowledge and self-discovery to bring understanding about how you are uniquely you—with your natural gifts and tendencies.

Getting to Know the Doshas

As you learn about each of the doshas, you'll probably strongly identify with one or two of them. There will be a certainty about it that only you can feel. *ding-ding!* That's when you know that it's you. Keep a rainbow mind-set and let the journey of self-discovery unfold as you go. You don't (and won't) know everything, and that's okay. Don't let the unknown trip you up; just keep going.

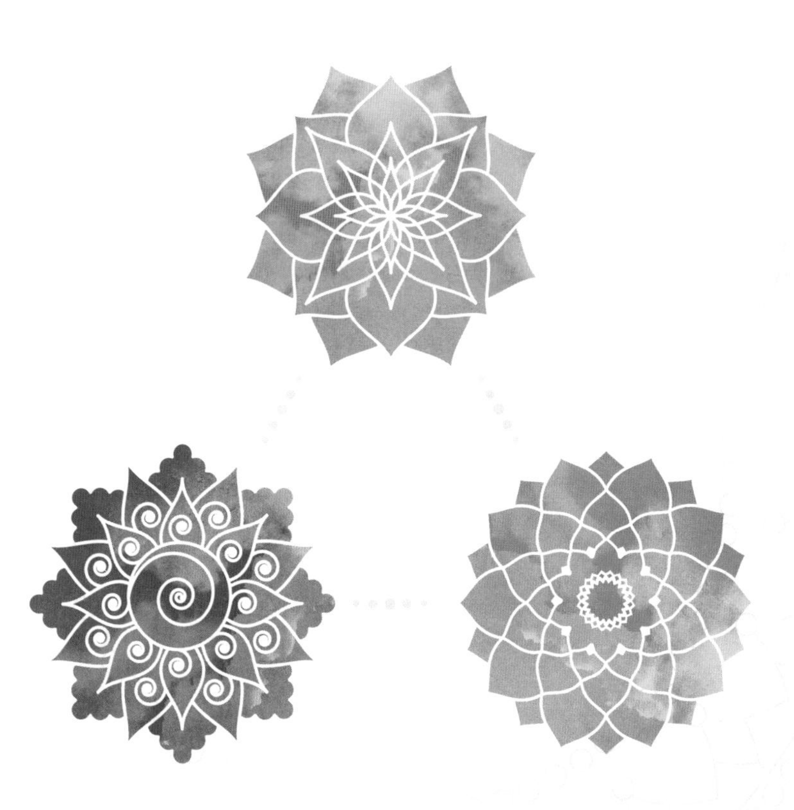

VATA DOSHA

Vata is known as the king of the doshas because pitta and kapha (the other two doshas) cannot move without it. Vata is involved in and influences almost everything. Vata's job is to create movement throughout the body and mind. People who have a lot of vata energy always feel like moving—it's hard for them to sit still.

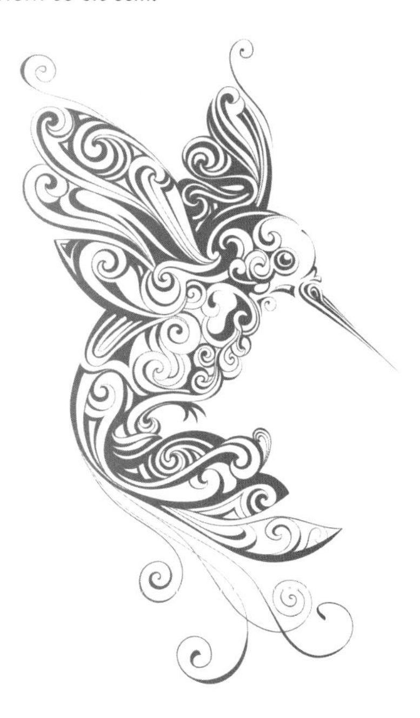

THE ENERGY OF MOVEMENT

Made of:
Space and air

Qualities:
Dry, light, cold, rough, subtle, initiates movement

Opposite qualities needed for balance:
Oily, heavy, warm, smooth, gross, stillness

Vata body: Light, slender build. Long, thin, oval features. Small eyes with little lashes. Irregular features (like crooked teeth or nose). Thin skin that browns in the sun and thin face. Dry, curly/frizzy hair. Dryness on the skin and eyes. They talk with their hands, very animated. They move fast, all the time. No matter what they eat, they stay thin.

Vata personality: They light up a room. Dramatic. Mood swings. Impulsive. Spontaneous. Creative. Expressive. Quick to change their minds or actions. Something is usually wrong or hurting. Tend to complain. Live in the future. Worried about the future. Insecure. Low confidence. They don't finish what they start. Full of ideas. Easily distracted. Hard to get them to stick to anything or stay in one place. They talk a lot and listen very little. Forgetful. Usually late. Often unreliable.

Signs of vata imbalance: Constipation, bloating, gas pains (they are a bit windy!), racing mind, worry, anxiety, panic, dryness, problems with the nerves, poor circulation, twitches/spasms, tightness, moving pain, weakness, depletion. Vatas go out of balance quickly (because they move fast like the wind), but can come back into balance quickly. The downside is that they can go out of whack again just as fast.

Vata has the most numerous imbalances because vata is involved in everything—and we live in a very vata-increasing world. We juggle a lot and our lifestyle tends to be fast-paced, overscheduled, and multitask-oriented. We often feel fast and ungrounded. So, if you feel a lot like a vata, that's pretty common. Vata energy in our environment or lifestyle has a strong influence over us, so we want to be mindful of balancing vata, especially because it has such an influence over the other two doshas as well.

Vata lifestyle recommendations: Warm weather, humidity or steam. Daily exercise to feel strong and grounded (walking, yoga, or weights). Warm oil massage on the skin. Create a reliable routine. Don't overschedule or overcommit. Do the same activities each day at the same time. Create space for stillness. Hang out with people who boost your confidence and bring you down to earth.

Vata diet recommendations: Warm, grounding, saucy/oily foods. Sweet and sour fruits, root vegetables, dairy, nuts, easy-to-digest grains, fats, and oils. A little meat sometimes. Oil is vata's number one food because vata is so dry. Resist the urge to eat eight meals a day. It is recommended that vata eat three meals at the same time each day. Limit dry, cold, or crunchy foods (like salads). Avoid brown rice and any grains that are high fiber because fiber is very dry and light. Also avoid peanuts. These foods all increase vata (hence constipation and gas) by making them colder, lighter, and drier, causing irregular and weak digestion.

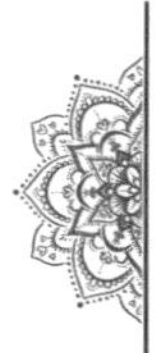

BALANCING ACT: *Slow down. Vatas love to move at the speed of light, but if they can learn to slow down their mind and body, they will find balance fairly easily! When they slow down, their mind can focus. And when their mind is focused, it influences the rest of their decisions and harmonizes their entire being.*

PITTA DOSHA

Pitta is the only dosha with the fire element, so anything that is heated, inflamed, red, acidic, or burning usually points to a pitta problem. Also, because pitta is the only dosha with fire, their digestion tends to be strong, because the fire element relates to our digestive fire (like increases like, so they have a healthy fire). Pitta helps transform and sort our food into our tissues and waste. Pitta's job is to transform things. Fire can nicely cook our food, transforming it into a meal for us, but fire can also burn things, and then we end up with charred potatoes on our plate. Pittas have strong intelligence because of their sharp quality. This intelligence and sharpness is what makes them great leaders—and why people love to follow them.

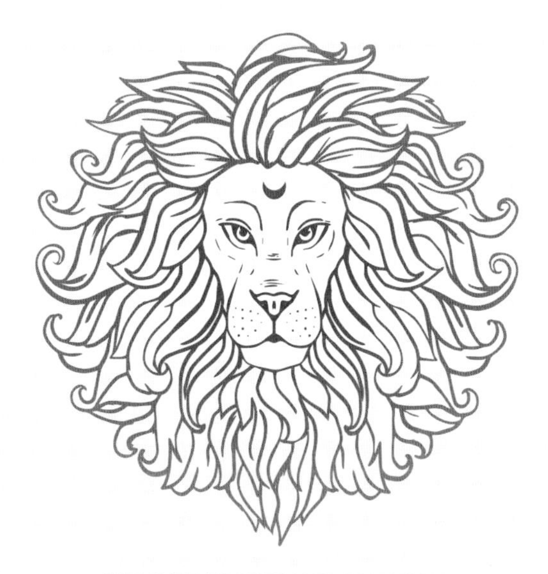

THE ENERGY OF TRANSFORMATION

Made of: Fire and water

Qualities: A little oily, sharp, hot, light, mobile, fluid

Opposite qualities needed for balance:
A little dry, dull, cool, heavy, stillness, sticky

Pitta body: Athletic, muscular, medium build. Sharp features that come to a point, like jaw, nose, or tongue. Eyes are sharp, piercing, and/or almond shaped. Wears contacts or glasses. Moles or freckles. Sensitive skin that burns in the sun. Straight, soft, silky hair. Graying, receding hairline, or balding.

Pitta personality: Sharp, to the point. Strong leader. Highly intelligent. Cerebral. Competitive. Witty. Lives in the present. Quick problem solver. Driven. Opinionated. Loves rules and may try to break them or make them work in their favor. Everything is a game. Entrepreneurial thinker. Debater. Persuasive. Organized. Mistakes jump out at them. Can't help but see all the details like, tpyos. Typos drive them nuts.

Signs of pitta imbalance: Inflammation or burning sensations anywhere. Skin problems like red rashes, blotchiness, or acne. Heartburn, sunburn, ulcers, acid reflux. Loose stools. Heated emotions like irritability, hostility, short temper, aggression, lack of patience.

Pitta takes a moderate amount of time to go out of balance and a moderate amount of time to come back into balance.

Pitta lifestyle recommendations: Cool weather, nothing too hot. Moderate exercise to create sweat and reduce stress levels (bike, swim, anything with wind in their face; do not exercise between 10 a.m. and 2 p.m.). Release control. Go with the flow. Stop working at night. Relaxation time. Hang with fun-loving friends who challenge you.

Pitta diet recommendations: Cooling foods like sweet fruits, vegetables, and dairy and grounding foods like nuts, healthy grains, and a little bit of oil. Fish or white meat is okay. Ghee is pitta's number one food because of its cooling quality. It is recommended that pitta eat three meals a day, with fruits for a snack. Limit spicy, sour, fermented, vinegary foods because these all increase heat in the body and agitate the mind.

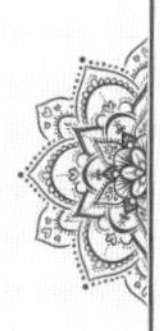

BALANCING ACT:

Pittas love to control situations and influence the outcomes, but pittas need to understand that they can't control it all. And in trying to do so, they will drive themselves (and others) crazy. Let go, pittas. The world will keep spinning even without your influence on all the details.

KAPHA DOSHA

Kaphas are the earthiest, most sturdy of the doshas. As the slowest and heaviest dosha, kapha's goal is to hold things together, providing structure and stability. They tend to be the healthiest of the three doshas because their mind is so steady; therefore, the body stays steady, in flow, and unstressed.

THE ENERGY OF LUBRICATION AND STRUCTURE

Made of: Water and earth

Qualities:
Oily, cold, heavy, slow, smooth/slimy, sticky, stable

Opposite qualities needed for balance:
Dry, warm, light, fast, rough, fluid, movement

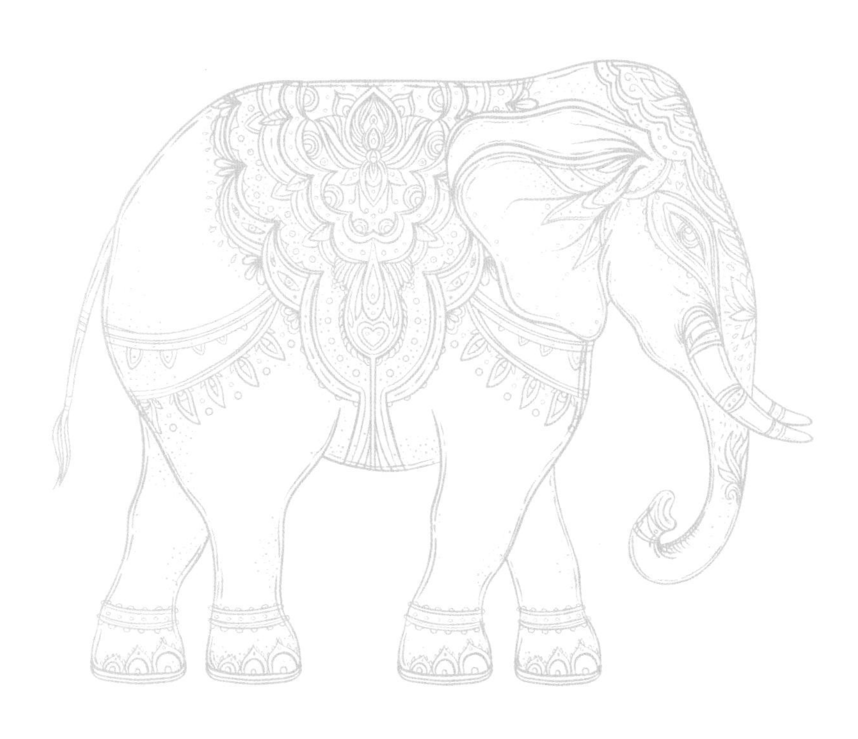

Kapha body: Large, strong build. Rounded and curvy features like round eyes with thick lashes, curvy hips, or barrel chest. Cool, thick skin. Thick, oily, wavy hair and thick hands. Have sweet faces, like an angel. Big strong teeth and bones.

Kapha personality: Nurturing. Tender. Patient. Consistent. Tolerant. Slow moving. Craves strong bonds. Emotionally strong yet sensitive. Loves to cook and host. Tends toward the lazy side. Can be very stubborn. Extremely generous. Doesn't like risk. Collects things. Finds it hard to let go or move on physically and emotionally. Lives in the past. Can hold grudges.

Signs of kapha imbalance: Weight gain. Lethargy. Cloudiness of mind. Cystic acne. Wet eczema. Allergies. Congestion. Diabetes. Edema. Greed. Envy. Intensely attached to material things. Out of the three doshas, kapha causes the least amount of health problems. It takes them a long time to get imbalanced because they are so mentally and physically sturdy. However, once a kapha gets imbalanced, it takes a lot of effort and a long time for them to get back to balance.

Kapha lifestyle recommendations: Dry heat. Sauna or the desert. Spiciness in food and life. Vigorous daily exercise to make you sweat (dance!). Try something new. Break up your routine. Adventure. Uplifting friends. Keep your physical space clean, devoid of clutter.

Kapha diet recommendations: Light, dry, and spicy foods. Fibrous fruits, vegetables, and light grains like quinoa, barley, and couscous. Limit or omit meats. Honey is kapha's number one food because it is heating and scraping. Since kapha is heavy and oily, the scraping quality helps kapha stay light and keep channels clear. Kaphas don't need a lot of food and do best with two meals a day. Limit rich, fried, salty, fatty, or oily foods because these all increase heaviness and oiliness—kapha has enough of that naturally.

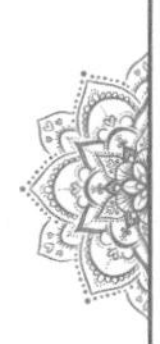

BALANCING ACT: *Release the past. Kaphas often cling to the past in their actions and thoughts, which hinders their forward motion and their forward progress. One of the best things kaphas can do is learn from the past, while taking inspired action in the present! Step forward, kaphas. The newness of today and tomorrow will dissolve old sad feelings of the past—release it and feel renewed.*

Which Dosha Do You Balance First?

Let's say you are a blend of doshas. Great, so how do you know which one to balance? Simply work on balancing the dosha that feels most like who you are right now, *today*.

 **TIP**: The best way for you to use this knowledge is to test and observe what feels best for your body and mind. We are all uniquely different! You will find your sweet spot of balance when you simply try some things.

Whatever you do, don't *stress* about your dosha. Your worries about perfection will create more problems than if you just feel into what you need, make a choice, and follow through. If you screw up, you'll feel a little junky and then you can just try something else.

You don't have to know everything about your dosha (even the best Ayurvedic doctors don't). But the important part is for you to realize that you are one of a kind and very simple diet and lifestyle guidelines should keep you in balance for the long term.

BRING IT TO LIFE

- Do any one (maybe two) of these doshas sound like you?
- Choose one diet or lifestyle change you can do to balance your dosha. Then, make a list of three to five more. When the first one becomes a habit, add the other changes one by one.
- Which one of these doshas sound like any of your coworkers or family members?
- How will you treat them differently based on what you know about them now?
- How will you use this knowledge to observe yourself and the people you love?
- If you are unsure about your dosha, the dosha test will help you. Find a link to my dosha test on page 143.

CHAPTER 3

It's All Your Fault

I know you are excited to learn about yourself, and you should be! But I have a little bad news. The word *dosha* literally means "fault." Think of the doshas as warning signs: "Warning! If you don't keep me balanced, I'm going to cause problems."

Each dosha has mental, emotional, and physical tendencies that are faults. Depending on our dosha, we will be naturally prone to certain faults. (Don't worry, it's not your fault. Ha. Sorry.) Use your knowledge of these not-so-awesome tendencies as your greatest challenge to master the things that are difficult or unnatural for you—these will require discipline. But that's okay because this is where your greatest powers for evolution, longevity, and lifelong balance lie.

Here's the kicker: Even when you think you have your health and balance aced, you *always* need to be mindful of getting pulled off course by your not-so-awesome dosha tendencies. As soon as you stop paying attention, the doshas will pull you out of balance. The doshas are in constant action and influence. Always. They show up again and again. Balancing them is a lifelong *practice*.

As you read about the tendencies, don't hold tight to whether or not it "belongs to your dosha." If something jumps out at you, pay attention because maybe that's something you need to work on. Your inner wisdom will know more than you think, and it will guide you to the right thing.

Trust that you know yourself better than anyone ever will.

The doshas all affect one another. So if one of the not-so-awesome tendencies totally sounds like you, work on it. It doesn't matter whether it's exactly your dosha or not because balancing that one tendency can help unravel other problems that are seemingly unrelated. In Ayurveda, everything is connected, so when you change one thing, you're likely to notice the benefits in many ways. If you resonate with one of the not-so-awesome tendencies, pay attention and work on it.

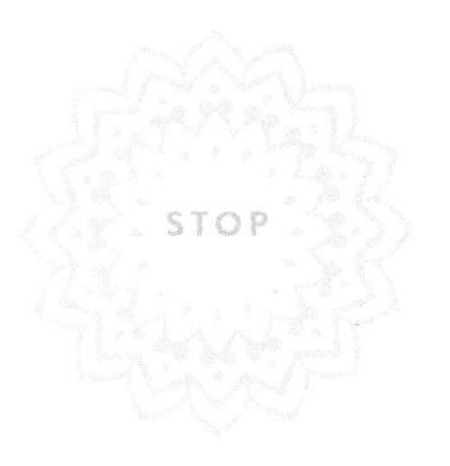

The Not-So-Awesome Vata Tendencies

Vatas are always on the move! Their nature is to instigate movement, so their mind and body might feel like they're constantly running. In a way, they are. Overall, vatas need to slow down and find their steadiness and structure. This theme of "steadiness" can be found in warming and heavy foods, a consistent routine, following through on your word, and getting regular sleep. Vata's strong nature to change like the wind can weaken their already sensitive confidence once they realize how many things they start but don't finish. So vatas, find your ground and consistency by overcoming these not-so-awesome vata tendencies.

TENDENCIES	DESCRIPTION	BALANCING ACT
Lacking focus and being easily distracted	Vatas can have a squirrely mentality. It's a constant challenge to keep their minds focused and adhere to finishing tasks.	Practice daily meditation. Play calming music or binaural beats to help your mind focus. Make sure you are warm enough—if vatas are cold, they can't concentrate.
Being a multitasker	Doing several things at once robs vata's already squirrelly focus, leading to the incompletion of things, which makes them then feel like failures and sinks their confidence.	Do one thing at a time. Complete it before you start on the next. Sticking to one thing and completing it will boost your confidence.

TENDENCIES	DESCRIPTION	BALANCING ACT
Eating multiple tiny meals each day	Vatas are notorious snackers of all things, especially of things dry and crunchy.	Eat three meals at the same time each day. Foods should be warm, saucy, and easy to digest. Vatas can't hold a lot of food, so if you often wake up hungry in the middle of the night, add a fourth meal, like a small bowl of rice around 8:30 p.m.
Having an inconsistent or no routine	They prefer spontaneity, but vatas need to practice a consistent routine every day.	Establish a good morning routine (see page 60) and do it every single day, without fail, without talking yourself out of it. A reliable routine gives vatas well-needed direction, structure, and peace of mind.
Worrying about the future	Distracting thoughts steal your concentration and hurt your confidence, causing indecision and lack of focus.	Practice daily meditation. **TIP:** Whenever you feel a little worried or uncertain, remember these words: *Relax, you are exactly where you are supposed to be, right now*. You are on a divine path and you can't ruin it. All your choices, whether seemingly good/bad, right/wrong, will roll up to give you the wisdom to become who you must be, in this lifetime. Relax.
Being flaky	Vatas tend to be late, cancel at the last minute, and change their minds like the wind, making them seem unreliable to others.	Stick to your word and follow through with your promises. Saying yes to fewer things will help you keep your commitments.

The Not-So-Awesome Pitta Tendencies

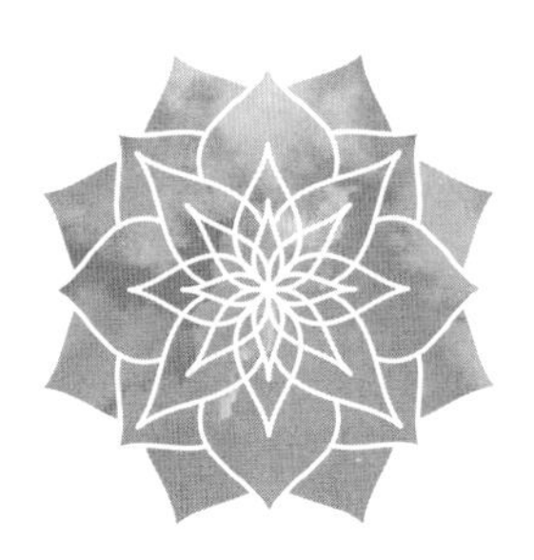

Since pittas run hot in their body and temperament; overall, they will need to stay cool and slow things down. This theme of "cool" covers both diet and lifestyle and includes cooling foods, cooling their temper, cooling their need for control, staying cool under stress, and even cooling their jets! Pittas love action and get super excited when they can influence outcomes in work or in life. However, their strong desire to drive, influence, and control can create unrealistic expectations of themselves and others, resulting in high stress levels. So, pittas, find your balance by overcoming these not-so-awesome tendencies.

TENDENCIES	DESCRIPTION	BALANCING ACT
Being controlling	Pittas would love to control everything if they could. But they can't control it all and will only drive themselves crazy if they try.	Let go and delegate. Choose to be hands-on only with the things that really matter to you. Then work on them with gusto, free of expectations, with full joy in the process. Learn to enjoy the process more than the outcome.
Being a workaholic	Pittas are good at what they do, but that doesn't mean they have to do it *all*. By maxing themselves out, they will eventually get cranky, resentful, or burn out.	Practice saying no (see page 111). Use your discernment and stop short of your maximum capacity so that you have time to reflect and rejuvenate.

TENDENCIES	DESCRIPTION	BALANCING ACT
Being a perfectionist	There's no such thing as perfection; everything has a flaw (or two, or six). If pittas stress about being perfect, they're in for a long, exhausting road ahead.	Take imperfect action. Share your gifts, even in their raw stages. Your bar is set so high that even your imperfections are better than most people's best efforts.
Having a sharp tongue	Pittas are naturally sharp and to the point, but their sharp words can cut others.	Be mindful of who you are talking to. Another pitta can handle your sharpness, but you need to buffer your delivery to vatas and kaphas, so you don't hurt or demotivate them.
Being a tough self-critic	Pittas have high expectations of others but are most critical of themselves. Pittas love a good challenge, but they may drive themselves to lengths they don't necessarily need to go to, beating themselves up in the process.	Be kind to yourself. You are doing your best. You are already awesome. You are enough.
Having a big appetite	Pittas have strong appetites, which can lead to overeating, especially when they are feeling stressed.	Reduce your salt intake (salt makes food tastier and can compel us to eat more) and eat more slowly. Eat happily and mindfully so you can taste the food and stop when you are satisfied instead of feeling full.

The Not-So-Awesome Kapha Tendencies

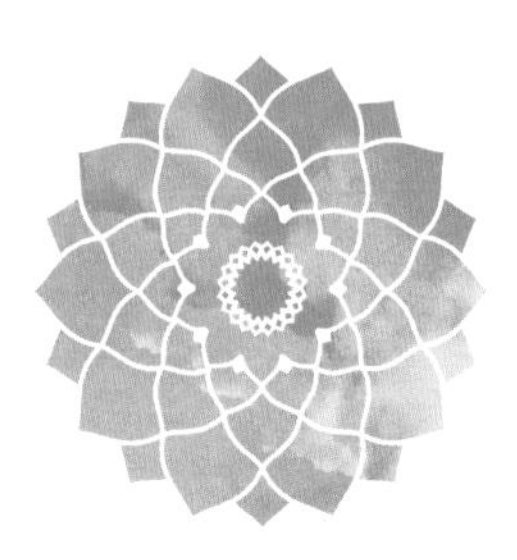

Kaphas are heavy and immobile, which is the area they need to counterbalance the most. Overall, they need to find their balance through lightness, heat, and mobility in their diet and lifestyle. They will feel best with spicy foods and a spicy life, and while they don't want to move, they will feel so happy after a good dance class or run/walk outdoors. Kaphas love security, reliability, and familiar comforts. However, in their desire to keep things familiar and safe, they can easily become immobile in thoughts and action, which hinders forward progress and often leaves them feeling "stuck." Kaphas, find your balance by overcoming these not-so-awesome tendencies.

TENDENCIES	DESCRIPTION	BALANCING ACT
Being a couch potato	Kaphas tend to be a bit lazy, so beware of their tendency to be immobile, creating heaviness in the body and the mind.	Move your body and work up a sweat daily. Do something fun like dancing so you stick with it and bring a buddy along with you for accountability!
Being stubborn	Kaphas are dang stubborn (that immobile thing), both physically and emotionally.	Be more flexible, whether it means saying yes to regular adventures or forgiving someone from your past. Becoming more mobile in your emotions will uplift and energize you.

TENDENCIES	DESCRIPTION	BALANCING ACT
Staying in your comfort zone	Feeling too comfortable is no good for kaphas because they will stay there and never move or evolve. Their lives will feel more enriched with challenges and discipline.	Make something with your hands, volunteer, clean a cluttered space, or move heavy things (like furniture).
Holding on to old emotions	Slow to change, kaphas are also slow at letting go of the past, especially heavy emotions and memories.	Let go of those old emotions—they happened way back then and are no longer serving you. You will feel lighter if you release them.
Eating too many sweets	Kaphas are drawn to sweets; however, rich or overly sweet foods create heaviness and sluggishness in the body, which weighs kaphas down physically, mentally, and emotionally.	Choose warm, light foods and make them spicy. A vegetarian or vegan diet is ideal for kaphas.
Collecting clutter	Kaphas tend to hold on to the crap. They are naturally attracted by an abundance of things, but over time, seeing and feeling the weight of all that stuff can weigh them down, creating physical and mental stagnation.	Clean out a closet, the garage, or any space that feels cluttered. When you get rid of physical stuff, your mind and your emotions will feel lighter.

BRING IT TO LIFE

- Jot down the dosha tendencies that sound most like you and choose one balancing act to work on immediately. Be mindful that you need to work on your not-so-awesome tendencies for the long term. They might always sneak up on you. But the great news is that now you'll be aware when they show up and you have fixes for them. Huzzah!

- What dosha tendencies do your loved ones have? Come up with three ways you can offer your loved ones more forgiveness and compassion based on what you've learned about their dosha tendencies and try to practice them when you interact with together.

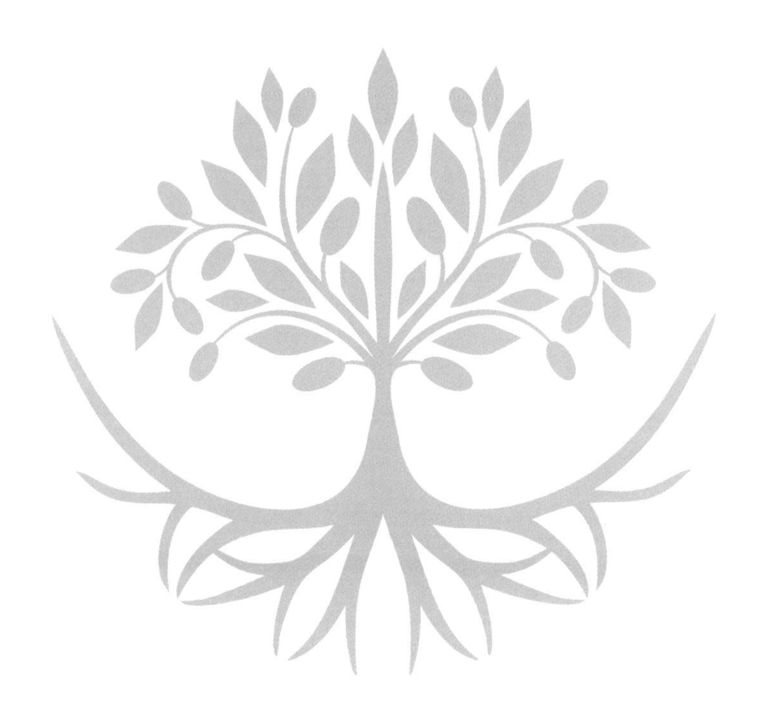

Congratulations! You have good roots now and you're ready to rise! In the next section, we dive into the details of routine, diet, and mind-set. Having strong tools to rise is the only way you can fully bloom!

Part 2

RISE

CHAPTER 4

Timing Is Everything

Now that you have strong roots with Ayurvedic foundations and knowledge of the doshas, you are ready for Part 2: Rise. Rising is the only way to reach new heights. When we rise, we change, we evolve, we get better, we may even impress ourselves when we realize we are stronger than we think we are! To rise, expect to apply new practices to your routine, diet, and mind-set. This is probably the hardest part because you have to put knowledge into action. You can get tripped up or worried about action, but if you keep a rainbow mind-set, knowing that any little step is a good step, you'll do just great.

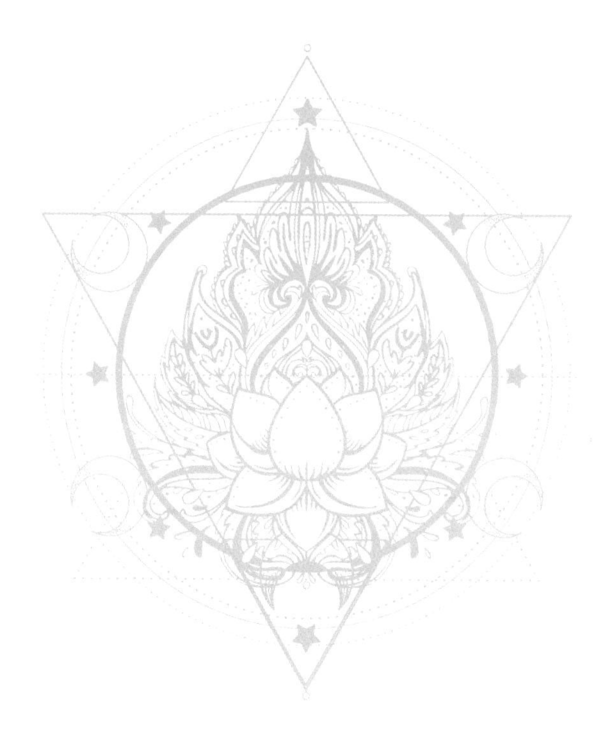

Daily Routine

The first way we rise is by creating a solid, daily routine.

When we want to make changes to our health, most of us usually aim straight for a diet and/or exercise routine first. It seems like the logical place to start because if we put the right foods in our bodies and move our bodies the right way, our bodies should change, right? Well, it depends.

What is usually missing in any diet or exercise regimen is timing. According to Ayurveda, timing is everything because nature has a rhythm! And nature's rhythm rules our daily routine.

The doshas govern time (and us), so going with a consistent rhythm has a big influence on our physical health, energy, and mind-set. When we go with the rhythm of nature, we feel more energetic, we get more done, we feel more in control of our day, and we get sick less often, too. A little realignment is so powerful that it can often be the remedy to heal and overcome health problems. Truth!

For instance, let's say you work out every day. On weekdays, you go for a run in the early morning in the dark. Although waking that early is not your favorite thing, it's the only time you have because of your work schedule, and honestly, you feel pretty awesome when it's done.

Weekends are another story. You happily sleep in and go for your morning run around 9 a.m., but you cannot figure out why your run feels heavier and more effortful. You breathe a little harder and your feet don't feel as light. You might even feel extra hot. Now, you may blame the wine from happy hour (actually a legit reason), but more than that, it's your timing.

If you were to do the same thing at two different times during the day, the way you feel doing it and the results would differ. Even if we do all the right things but at the wrong time, we actually might end up feeling worse. It can feel as if you're trying to swim upstream. This can affect your sleep, your productivity, your weight, your energy, and more.

Adjusting our daily routines to nature's clock is a game changer! A little realignment goes a long way. When you start doing the right things at the right time, you will take your energy, your health, and your productivity to another level. So, let's make the day easy on you and sort out your daily routine.

The Timing of Digestive Fire

Because everything in Ayurveda is connected, the rhythm of your daily routine directly links to your proper function of digestion. Eating at the right time, in the right quantity, is essential because not digesting our food well is one of the main causes of health problems. So before we even go into the times of day to do things, let's do a quick introduction of how digestive fire works, first.

In Ayurveda, it is said that our digestive fire burns behind our belly button and in Sanskrit that is called *agni* (UG-knee). Agni is responsible for digesting, absorbing, and assimilating our food. When agni functions properly, we digest food well, think clearly, poop regularly, and have strong immunity. When agni doesn't function well, the food is not digested all the way and we end up with old food junk hanging around in the body, which turns into a sort of toxin. From there, the toxins make their way into weak tissues, causing physical and mental problems.

On the other hand, when agni functions well, we stay pretty darn healthy because digestion directly influences everything else.

Now that you know what agni is, here's how it functions. The strength of agni rises and sets with the sun. Going back to the macrocosm/microcosm root, the sun is the giant fire and agni is our mini fire (macrocosm/microcosm), so the health of our digestion depends a lot on *when* we are eating and in what quantity. At sunrise, agni is not very strong because neither is the sun—it's low on the horizon and therefore agni is low within us too. By around noon or midday, the sun is at full strength and so is agni. At dinnertime, the sun is setting and agni is also starting to lose its power for the day. In a nutshell, for two meals out of three, agni is low.

We will go into more detail, but it's important to understand agni's rhythm during the day.

Now that you're equipped with a little knowledge of agni, let's dive into the rhythm of the Ayurvedic daily routine.

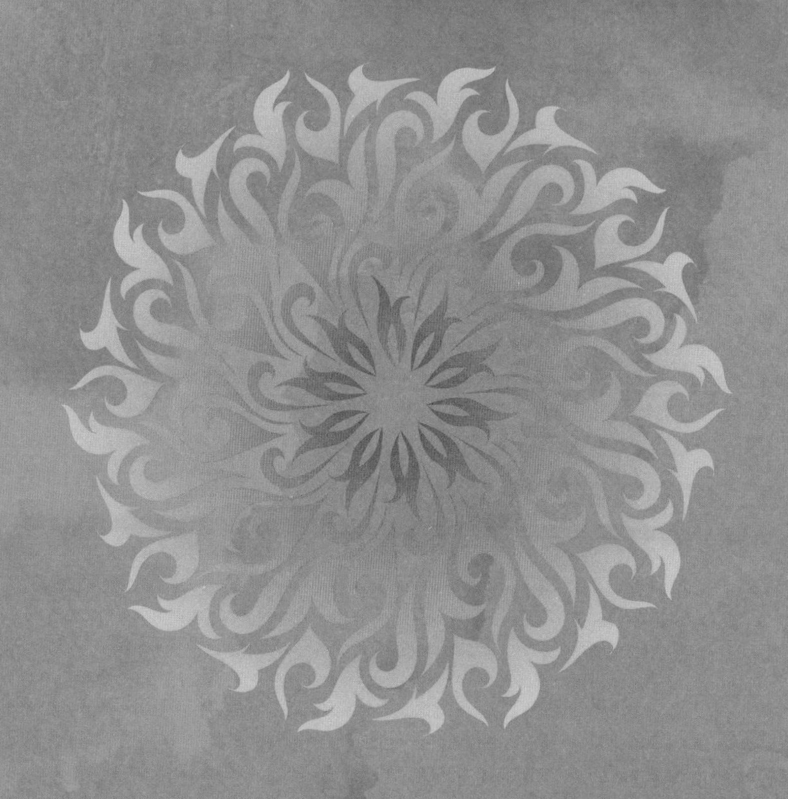

A malfunctioning agni
is the root cause for most
diseases and imbalances.

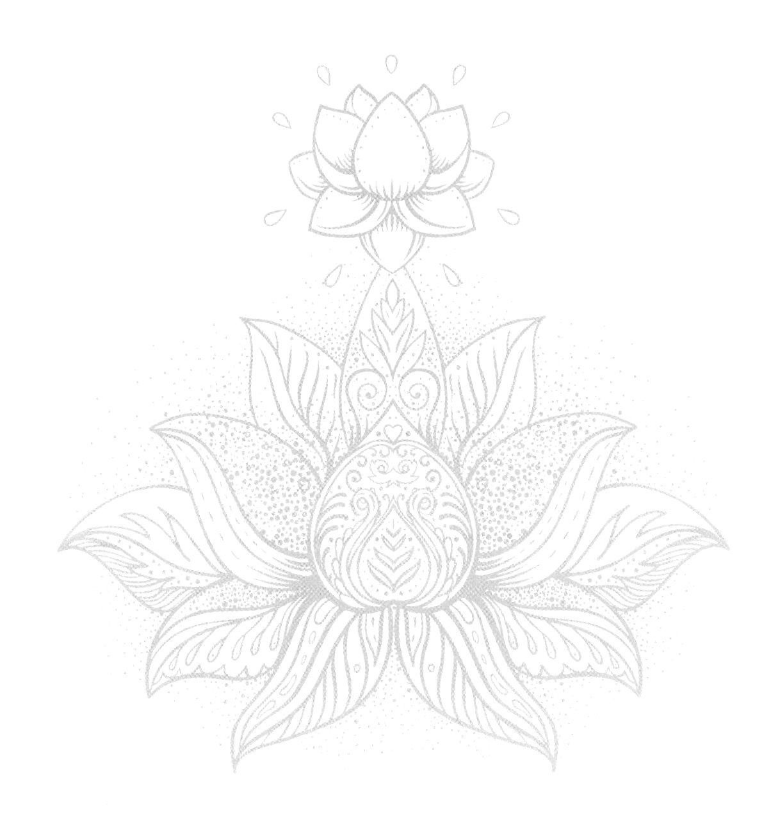

Daytime

The doshas are constantly changing even in nature, but I've ballparked the time frames for you, so if you stick to these guidelines, you'll do just fine. In the following pages, you'll learn how the doshas and their qualities govern the time of day.

SUNRISE TO 10 A.M. IS KAPHA TIME

Kapha time is slow and heavy energy. It's an excellent time for production and powering through work that doesn't need too much thinking. It's not a great time for strategy or creativity. Do the bulk of your work here and the rest of the day will feel like it flows easily. Your normal routine may be to sift through emails, leisurely sip coffee, gab with coworkers, and putz around because you're "not a morning person." But resist that urge. Get your stuff done and do the heavy lifting at the right time. You will get so much done between 7:30 a.m. and 10 a.m. you'll surprise yourself. You will feel so accomplished early, which will motivate you throughout the day and will give you extra time to play later!

KAPHA MORNING PITFALL #1:

Eating a cold, goopy breakfast.

Kapha is cold and heavy, and agni is low. Using our root of "like increases like," if we add something cold, goopy, and heavy to a tiny fire, what happens? Yep, the fire goes out. That's not what we want.

Balancing Act: Have a small, warm breakfast to act as kindling, so that agni grows to be strong by lunch. Agni is low and weak in the morning, so if you have cold food or too much quantity of food, you'll weaken agni further. Yogurt and smoothies are not advised at this time because they are cold and raw, with no fire (heat!) element in them, so they could dampen agni first thing in the morning and it will have a hard time growing to full strength to digest lunch. It's also okay to skip breakfast if you're not hungry. Over time, this habit could cause cloudiness of mind, lethargy, poor digestion, or low immunity.

KAPHA MORNING PITFALL #2:

Having no morning agenda and wasting power time.

Kapha is a follower, so when we sit down at our desks, it's essential to have our morning (or day!) plan already laid out for us. Then it will be easy to follow the plan and get it done. Otherwise, we will daydream, wander, and putz our power time away simply because we don't have a plan or clear direction.

Balancing Act: Make your morning task list the previous day so it's waiting for you in the morning. Then all you have to do at kapha "follower" time is follow your list.

10 A.M. TO 2 P.M. IS PITTA TIME

Pitta time of day is all intellect, organizing, sorting, and analyzing. Use this time for strategy meetings, talking out big ideas, or problem solving. And eat lunch as your biggest meal of the day because agni is strongest here. Pitta is the only dosha with the fire element in it, so around noon, the sun, agni, and pitta are all in alignment—all three fires!—and it's the strongest our agni will be all day. Take advantage of this fire power and have lunch as your biggest meal.

PITTA MIDDAY PITFALL: Skipping lunch.	
This is the one of the biggest mistakes I see in busy people's routines. We are usually so busy cranking out work and going from meeting to meeting, who has time to stop for lunch? Right. Well, if you skip lunch, you'll be starving in the afternoon, will go looking for snacks (sweets and convenience food), and you will likely overeat at dinner because you haven't eaten anything good all day. Overeating at dinner as a habit leads to weight gain, sleep disturbances, digestive problems, and low immunity. Skipping lunch can cause all this!	**Balancing Act:** Eat lunch! Agni is strongest this time of day, so use its power to fuel you throughout the day. This way, you won't be hungry in the afternoon, and instead of losing your energy and chasing shiny objects, you'll be able to maintain your focus. You also most likely won't overeat at dinner.

2 P.M. TO SUNSET IS VATA TIME

Vata time is in the afternoon, so if you get antsy around 2 p.m. or notice an energy slump, you are being affected by vata energy. You know how it goes. You might want to go get a coffee, distract your coworkers, or do high kicks and jumping jacks in the office (just me?) because vata is the energy of movement, which sparks ideas and makes us want to move! This is an optimal time for brainstorms, creativity, idea sharing, meetings (I used to have walking meetings outside), or a workout! This is also the perfect time to write out your task list for the morning because vata time will spark so many ideas, including things you want to do, things you must do, and things you can't forget to do. Write them down and then knock out the list in the morning when it's kapha time to maximize your productivity.

VATA AFTERNOON PITFALL #1:

Frittering time.

Your mind and body will likely feel restless at this time, so instead of letting your mind go on autopilot by wasting time or making poor decisions, use the energy of movement to your advantage.	**Balancing Act:** Go to recess! Take a walk outside or squeeze in a short workout if you can. Vata energy is making you want to move, so go with it. If you try to stifle it, you'll figure out unproductive ways to move or distract yourself, so you may as well get off your tushy, take a nice break, and move your body.

VATA AFTERNOON PITFALL #2:

Mindlessly snacking or grabbing another coffee.

Snacking aggravates vata because it causes irregularity in digestion. If you are already "irregular," this might be why.	**Balancing Act:** Adhere to meals at the right time and quantity, consistently, and your digestion will improve. Skip the coffee—it's vata-aggravating.

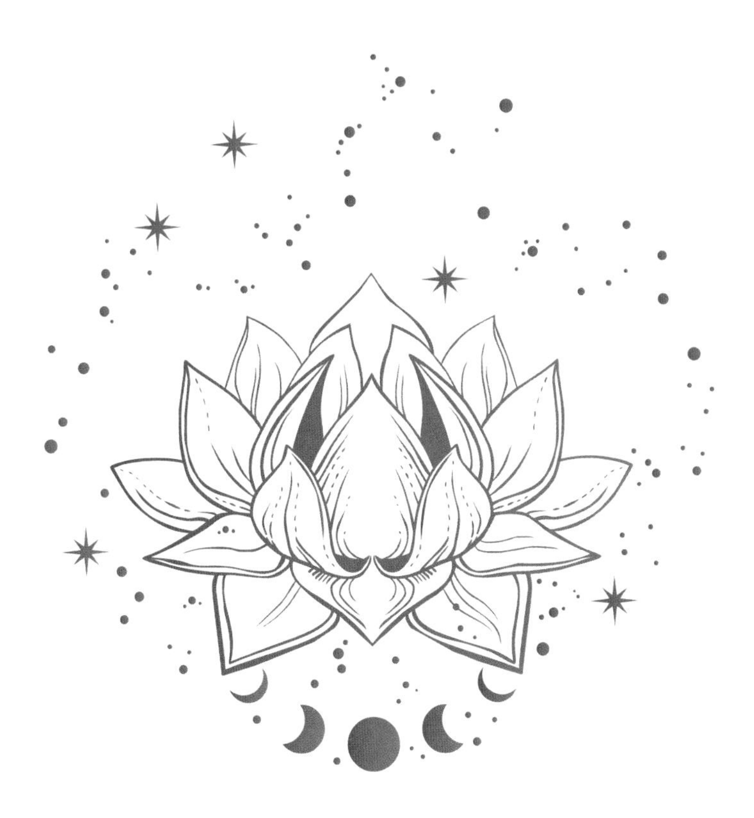

Nighttime

SUNSET TO 10 P.M. IS KAPHA TIME

Since kaphas are all about love, peace, and harmony, this is the time to be with family, eat a small dinner, and relax. Enjoy this time. Feel good about what you accomplished today. This time is *not* for working more and pushing through. There's a time when we have to just be done working or we will burn ourselves out. The other neat thing about this time frame is because kapha energy is heavy and slow it will put us to sleep easily. It's slow, cozy time that preps us for a good night's sleep.

KAPHA EVENING PITFALL: Eating too much quantity of food at dinner.	
Because the sun is going down, agni is just not strong this time of day and the food will stay undigested until morning. If this is habitual, it can cause weight gain, a cloudy mind, and overall fatigue.	**Balancing Act:** Have a small dinner. Dinner should be about half the size of lunch. The exact food doesn't matter as much as the quantity. Don't eat enough to feel full; eat enough so you are no longer hungry.

TIP: Kapha time rules two out of three meals! Kapha is slow and heavy. Two small meals and one large meal is the rhythm. If you make only this one change, you will arrive at a healthy weight for you and your daily energy will improve.

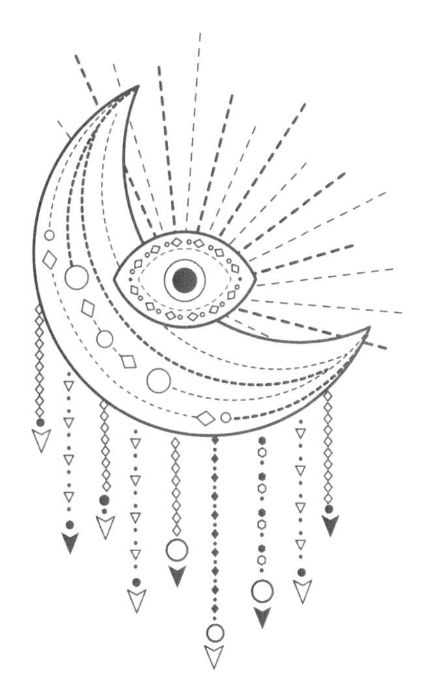

10 P.M. TO 2 A.M. IS PITTA TIME

Here's where the magic happens, and pitta does all of the processing from the day. You should be in bed at this point. Pitta will transform and digest all your food, emotions, and thoughts from the day. So, if you are not sleeping by 10 p.m., you've crossed into pitta time and you'll probably be up for a while. Here's why: pitta creates what feels like a "second wind" and you'll start doing pitta-esque things that feel very important, like deep cleaning the fridge, reorganizing your spreadsheet for holiday card recipients, and color-coding the clothes hanging in your closet while starting a donation pile.

Pitta will do the sorting and transforming whether you are sleeping or awake—you just happen to be awake for the gong show and so you act accordingly. This may feel good because you are "most productive at night," but being a habitual night owl will likely lead to long-term sleep problems that can affect immunity and cause vata-type problems because you are not getting the amount of sleep you need. Being a night owl goes against the flow of nature's clock.

Agni needs a long fast each night so it can fully digest all the food you ate that day. If you are a midnight snacker and choose to eat at this time, it's a fast track to weight gain.

PITTA NIGHTTIME PITFALL: Staying up past 10 p.m.	
Almost everybody I know who has sleep problems has had a habit of staying up too late at some point in their life and now they have sleep troubles, which leads to other problems as well.	**Balancing Act:** Get to bed by 10 or 10:30 p.m. at the latest or pitta will keep you awake! Get your booty to bed on time. You'll likely feel sleepy before 10 p.m. anyway, because kapha energy is slowing you down, so go with it and use that feeling of heaviness to hit the sack for a good night's sleep.

BREAKING THE RULES:

This late night pitta time will help you get stuff done. If you have a big project due, this time is a secret dose of magic. And oh yes, I've used it to my advantage (pittas like to make rules work in their favor, remember?). When I wrote my first book, I was a new mom, had a demanding day job, and had a three-hour daily commute. The only time I had to write was between 9 p.m. and 1 a.m., so that's what I did. I stayed up late for one or two nights and then would fall on my face at 8 p.m. for two nights to rebalance myself. Then repeat. It was short-lived, but it totally worked. You can do some of your best work at this time, but just don't make it a habit!

2 A.M. TO SUNRISE IS VATA TIME

Vata is present in the wee hours of the morning before sunrise. This is when we are connected to the subtle energy of nature and our highest self. This time is ideal for waking because when you rise in the energy of vata, the energy of movement will carry you throughout the day—like a nice energetic wind in your sails. This time is also ideal for working out—your workouts will feel effortless and the best feeling is when it's 7 a.m. and your workout is complete. It's like you already won the day. This is also a great time for studying because you will have time to remember what you learned during the day. If you study at night, pitta will process out the new information during sleep.

VATA EARLY MORNING PITFALL:

Waking when the sun is up.

Yes, you read that correctly. Waking when the sun comes up is a pitfall because If you wait until the sun is up, you'll be rising in the energy of kapha (slow, heavy). Kapha makes it harder to get out of bed and you'll have a groggy start and potentially a groggy day.	**Balancing Act:** Rise in the dark. Even fifteen minutes before sunrise will do, as long as it's dark out. As a bonus, waking up this early will make you good and tired to get to bed by 10 p.m. And there you go: two birds, one stone.

Often, it's only a matter of a fifteen- or thirty-minute time shift that will make *all* the difference in how we feel each day and how we build our diet and lifestyle habits. Don't be fooled—seemingly minor adjustments can have a major impact. Trust that even small changes will make a big difference. We will digest food better, produce better work more efficiently, have sharper focus, sleep better, even arrive at a weight that's right for us. Remember, nature is our home and our guiding force—when we become part of its schedule and flow with it, our lives rebalance and feel more in flow quite easily.

TIP: Realigning your day to do the right things at the right times will help you grow and change, fast! The hardest part will be actually *doing the practices*. Commit to one change at a time so that you are successful. And see chapter 6 to anticipate your missteps.

BRING IT TO LIFE

- How is your schedule already in alignment with the daily routine? Check the book extras on page 143 for a downloadable daily routine.
- How is your schedule out of alignment with the daily routine? Choose one or two realignments to change in your schedule.

CHAPTER 5

Eat Happily and Intuitively

In this chapter, you'll rise up when you discover a new level of nutrition! Here's something that may surprise you: food is not necessarily the most important part of our overall nutrition. In Ayurveda, *how* we eat is just as important as *what* we eat. In this chapter, you'll need to use your rainbow mind-set and get ready for a brand-new perspective on food.

In Ayurvedic nutrition, there are no diets. No measuring, no constricting. Nothing is off-limits. You are simply aware of foods that make you feel good and those that don't. When you choose the right foods, you feel light in your body, your digestion works well, you poop well *high five*, and your mind is clear. You have total peace and enjoyment because you are choosing food that works for you.

So often, in our attempts to eat "correctly," we end up confused or doubtful. Here we are just trying to do the right thing, but in trying to do so, it can cause more stress, which takes the love and enjoyment out of food! Love, enjoyment, and gratitude are key ingredients to digesting food well.

Let's take away some of that confusion and step into a more intuitive, joyful approach to eating.

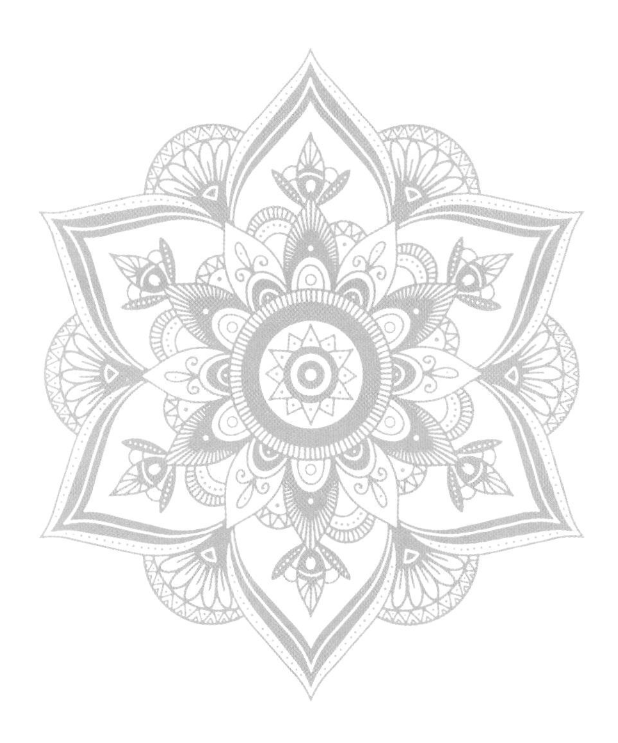

Calories Do Not Exist

For real, Ayurveda does not have calories. If we don't have calories, how do we know whether we've eaten enough or too much? Ah! Instead, we use a more intuitive approach by paying attention to real hunger, making sure we have plenty of variety, and choosing foods that are high-quality. We check in with ourselves, often. If we pay attention, we already know the right amount of food that feels best for our bodies. We do! We don't have to rely on someone else giving us a number to hit for our food; we know ourselves better than anyone, and if we tap in, we will know when we've eaten too much or too little. And then we can adjust if needed. Remember, walk the middle path. Variety is where we find balance—too much or too little of any certain type of food will cause imbalance. Besides, if the main goal is to eat happily, how can we fully enjoy our food if we spend our time counting or judging it? Let us not create restrictions or judgements and, instead, let's love the food while eating the right amount for our unique selves.

Wait for the hunger burn. In addition to eating at the right time, as per the daily routine, the best guide to know when to eat is to wait until you feel a hunger burn. That "burning" hunger sensation is actually agni (fire, burn!) letting you know it's ready for food. If you have not paid much attention to when you feel hungry and when you don't, this will be a powerful practice to start. Your body tells you what it needs all the time, and when you honor its signals, you will intuitively know how to care for it. Impactful learning and healing happen when you actually tap into what your body needs!

Not too much quantity. If you refer back to chapter 4, you'll notice that two out of the three meals happen in kapha time, which is slow and heavy. So, you might need way less food than you think you do. We have grown accustomed to large quantities, so let's use this as knowledge to adjust portion sizes that support the body's digestion and proper building of tissues. Otherwise, we are just being driven by our taste buds (which is just ego, btw), which can cause us to overeat.

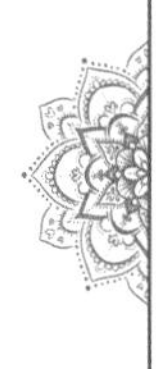

BALANCING ACT: *If you feel like you are eating too much in quantity, have only one plate or bowl of food, no seconds. Dinner should be pretty small, sometimes even a piece of fruit will do the trick (all the pittas just cracked up laughing) and you're good until morning. But as always, you'll have to test things out to find what works for you.*

There Is No Such Thing as Good or Bad Food

Rainbow mind-set does not see foods as good or bad. In Ayurveda, there is no such thing, because any food can be nectar and any food can be poison, depending on who's taking it. There's the "it depends" rule again. For example, let's say a pitta person with strong agni has a salad for lunch and they feel just fine. A vata person with weak agni may have that same "healthy" salad and get bloated. If the vata person ignores these signs and chooses salad on a regular basis, they could end up with larger digestion problems like constipation. So even the "good" foods can cause problems for certain people. Again, there is no such thing as good or bad food, only foods that you can digest well and those that you can't. The most important thing about food is how we digest it—and everybody is different.

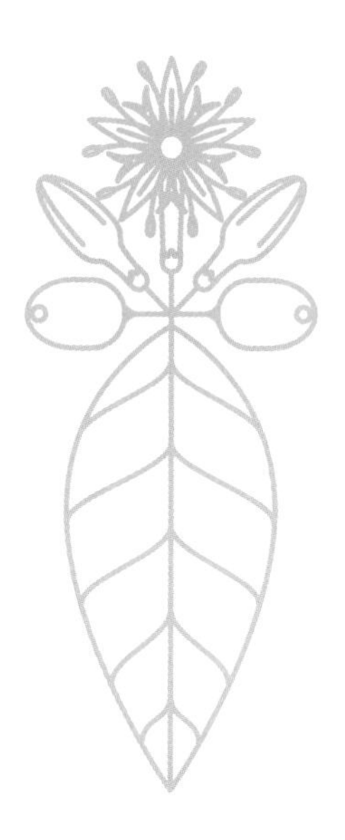

Choose high-quality food. While there are no good or bad foods, there are definitely high-quality and low-quality foods. High-quality foods build high-quality tissues to create our physical body and build good immunity. They also give us a higher quality of mind (more in chapter 6). If you put low-quality foods into your body, it will create a lower quality of mind. If you choose low-quality foods often, you'll notice a downward spiral into the land of negative talk and beliefs. Motivation and energy levels may go down, while doubts and pessimism increase. If you notice you are more negative, doubtful, or irritated, take a look at what you are eating because you may need to make a change.

We want to frequently eat what happily grows, like fruits, veggies, and grains, because these foods contain good prana (vital life force or life energy). The closer the food is to nature, the higher quality the food will be because a) it's higher in prana and b) our body will be able to recognize, assimilate, and digest that food better. These foods were created by the earth, the sun, and the rain (elements!), so love 'em up and eat 'em often! Eat these foods more often than not and it will keep your mind, mood, and thoughts healthy and on the positive side. Eating food from nature is not "taking the fun out of food"; it's about getting the fullest, highest nourishment out of the meal—because food is our fuel and the building blocks for our entire mind and body!

So in a nutshell, high-quality foods are foods that you can easily identify: you know where they come from or how they're grown, and you can pronounce all the ingredients (if they have a label). High-quality foods include fruits, vegetables, grains, some dairy, herbs, spices, and maybe some meats, depending on their source. Having meals with high-quality ingredients is the best way to create a high-quality mind and body.

Low-quality foods include highly processed foods, frozen, stale, canned, modified or manipulated, and of course "mystery" foods. A mystery food is anything that isn't clear on what it is or how it's made. A good clue is the items that misspell their main ingredient like, "cheez puffz" or "vegan chick'n stix." (I still don't understand how anything vegan can or would want to be called chicken . . . I digress.) When we can't identify where the food came from, nor can we pronounce or understand the ingredients on the label, it's a low-quality food. Low-quality foods don't have any prana! Remember, prana is our life energy, our vital life force. If the food doesn't have life energy, you won't either.

Reduce the hot dogs, squeeze cheese, sodas . . . I think you get my drift. This isn't news to you. You already know you need to make good food choices, but this helps you understand why: because foods that are far away from the source of nature—and you're made of nature—won't be digested well, and these foods will build a low-quality body, mind, and spirit, which creates low-quality mood, decisions, emotions, and mind-set—and that stuff is everything!

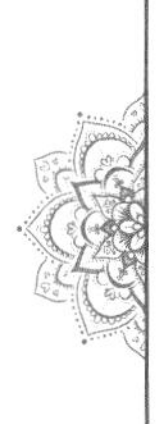

BALANCING ACT: *If you eat high-quality foods 80 to 90 percent of the time, you win! Use the 10 to 20 percent to enjoy the occasional cupcake, cheese puffs, and glass of wine because those are treats and part of life's enjoyment and celebration!*

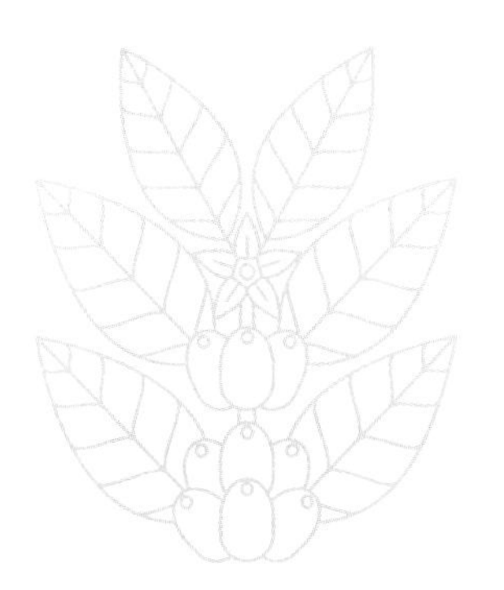

Variety is where to find joy and balance. Variety is the key to a balanced nutrition without having to overthink or stress about it. If you have the same ol' brown foods over and over, you are missing out on tastes, spices, and nutrients found in a variety of foods. For example, maybe you are stuck in a rut of eating meals like this: chicken and rice, refried beans and rice, or meat n' potatoes, chicken sandwich with fries, or chicken with pasta. These are pretty commonplace meals, but they lack color (all beige or brown!), vibrancy, and good, life-giving prana. You'll eat happier when you see the nice colors decorating your plate! As a beautiful bonus, when food smells good, looks good, and has nice variety, it is pleasing and satisfying to the mind. Peace in the mind creates balance of the entire body, and so when we use food the right way, food becomes good medicine.

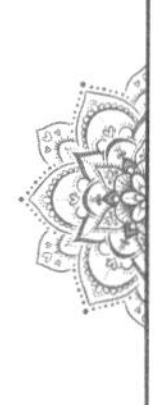

BALANCING ACT: *Double-check your plate and meals to include yummy variety, not just carbs and protein; also bring in the bitter, astringent tastes from greens and veggies as well as a little pungent spice. Use wonderful spices like mint, basil, cilantro, cinnamon, black pepper, salt, the list goes on! Celebrate the variety! Walking the middle path is where we find our balance, even in food. Choose some carbs, some veggies, some fruits, and some meat if you need it.*

Eat in a good mood. It doesn't always matter exactly what you eat, but it always matters *how* you eat. It is absolutely crucial to eat in a happy mood. Not a stressed mood. Not a crabby mood. Not a depressed mood. We digest emotions just as we digest food. No matter how organic, how fresh, how expensive, how pure the food is, if our mind is not in a happy place when eating, we won't digest the food well.

We must warm the food
with our spirit
so our body will accept
the food.

Food is important, but not *the* most important, and should never be a source of stress or worry. But many of us do worry, right? Like, "Is this the right food for me? I'm afraid I will overeat. I'm afraid I'll make bad choices. Is this food bad? Is this type of food too carby, too sugary, too meaty, too whatevery?"

We sometimes put judgments and fears into our food before it even hits our mouth. These fearful and worrisome messages from the mind get transmitted throughout the body (mind, body, and spirit are all connected, remember?) and we can end up not digesting *any* food well just because we have so much worry around eating. Whatever mental beliefs or challenges you have with food—whether confusion, fear, or inconvenience—those alone could be causing poor digestion or imbalance.

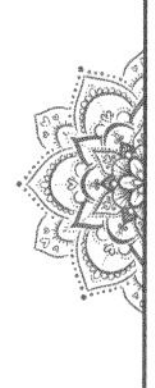

BALANCING ACT: *Eat happy. Generate a positive mood by calming your mind with some breathwork, a short meditation, or moving your body with a short walk, yoga series, or workout. You don't even need to be an ace at your own nutrition yet; all you have to do is be happy and grateful for whatever you are eating in this moment.*

All positive emotions surround the meal because we digest our emotions and thoughts just as we digest our food. If our mind thinks our food is "bad" in any way, our body will respond accordingly with digestive problems or other imbalances—simply because we put fear or judgment in the food. The food doesn't matter nearly as much to your nutrition as your mood does.

You need higher food. If you struggle with weight, food issues, out-of-control cravings, or obsessions, this next part might completely change your life. If you feel a tight cling to food and you're not sure why, you might be missing higher food. What is higher food?

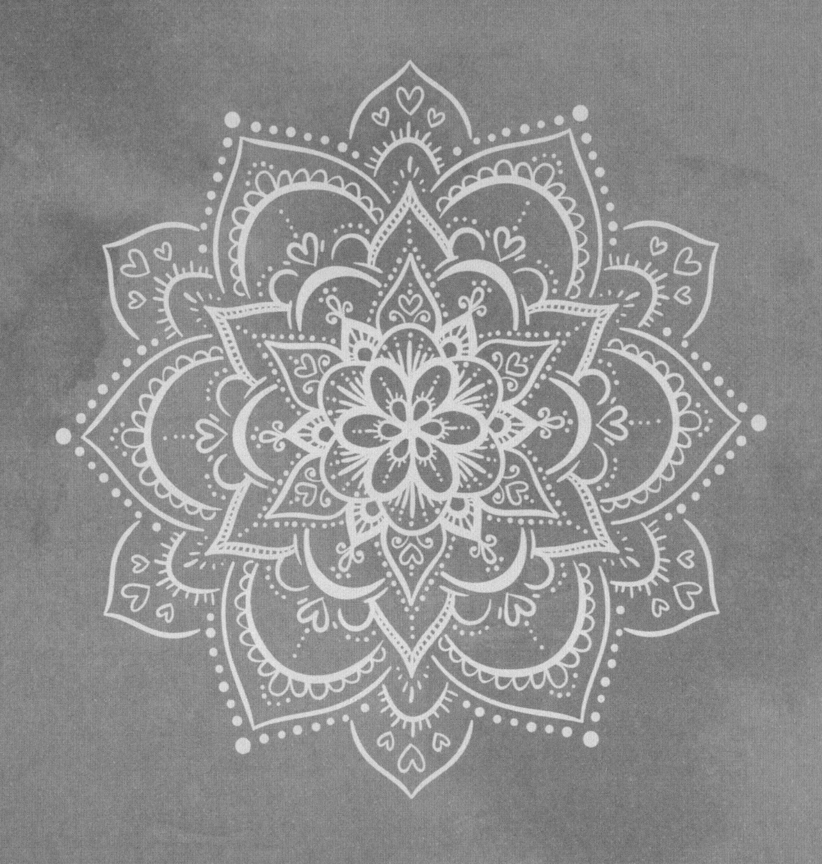

Higher food is love.
Love of others.
Love of self.
Love of adventure.

When we feel void of love, we go seeking to fill that void with other things, and for many people, it's food. Food is tasty. The sense of taste is ruled by the ego. When food is tasty, the ego says, "I want more of that!" and if it's habitual, over time we can find ourselves relying heavily on food for entertainment, emotional comfort, and social connection.

But here's the empowering part. When you realize that you are only using food because you are missing higher food, you can make a new choice. Reach for higher food like love, adventure, spending time in nature, and learnings something you are passionate about. These new habits will help dissolve the old obsessions, addictions, and worries. Cravings will get smaller because your focus on receiving and emitting love has gotten bigger.

For example, when you first start dating someone you're crazy about, what happens? You lose your appetite! You're so full up on love thinking about this new sparkly person that you forget to eat, don't need to eat, whatever, what's my name again? The love and happy feelings are keeping you full.

The same thing happens when we are fully engaged in a project or an activity that we might get lost in. It could be anything like writing, painting, building, knitting, gardening, or playing with puppies, and we "forget" to eat. When we are so engrossed in something we love, we just don't need a lot of food!

Higher food or love is much more filling and potent than any morsels we can put into our mouths.

What about cravings? When should we listen to a craving? How do we know whether our body needs it, whether it's a special treat, or whether we are going overboard? Simply ask yourself: Is it reasonable? If you want a treat, have it. You know when you are being unreasonable. Two or three Girl Scout cookies are reasonable. The whole box, not reasonable.

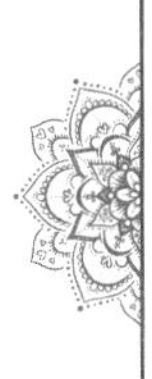

BALANCING ACT: *Are you missing higher food? The cravings for food might simply be a calling for higher food. Build space between you and the craving. Do an activity that nourishes your mind or soul first. Then, if you still have the craving, go ahead and have it, just be reasonable about it.*

Here's the thing: We *do* crave foods that balance us, even if they don't seem like it. This is where the intuitive part of eating comes in. For example, when we ladies have our menstrual cycles, sometimes we crave chocolate. The blood is ruled by pitta (which is hot), so cravings like chocolate make sense because the sweet is cooling.

For instance, increased vata will crave foods that are light, dry, crunchy, and cold. These foods will keep increasing vata. Increased pitta will crave spicy, salty, and oily foods, which will keep increasing pitta. Increased kapha will crave foods that are rich, extra sweet, salty, or heavy, which will keep increasing kapha. So, do self-checks often and if you have over-the-top cravings for the things that don't balance your dosha, replace those with the right foods that do balance your dosha, which we will talk about next.

TIP: The next time you go grocery shopping, make it a point to add one new and balancing food item to your grocery list.

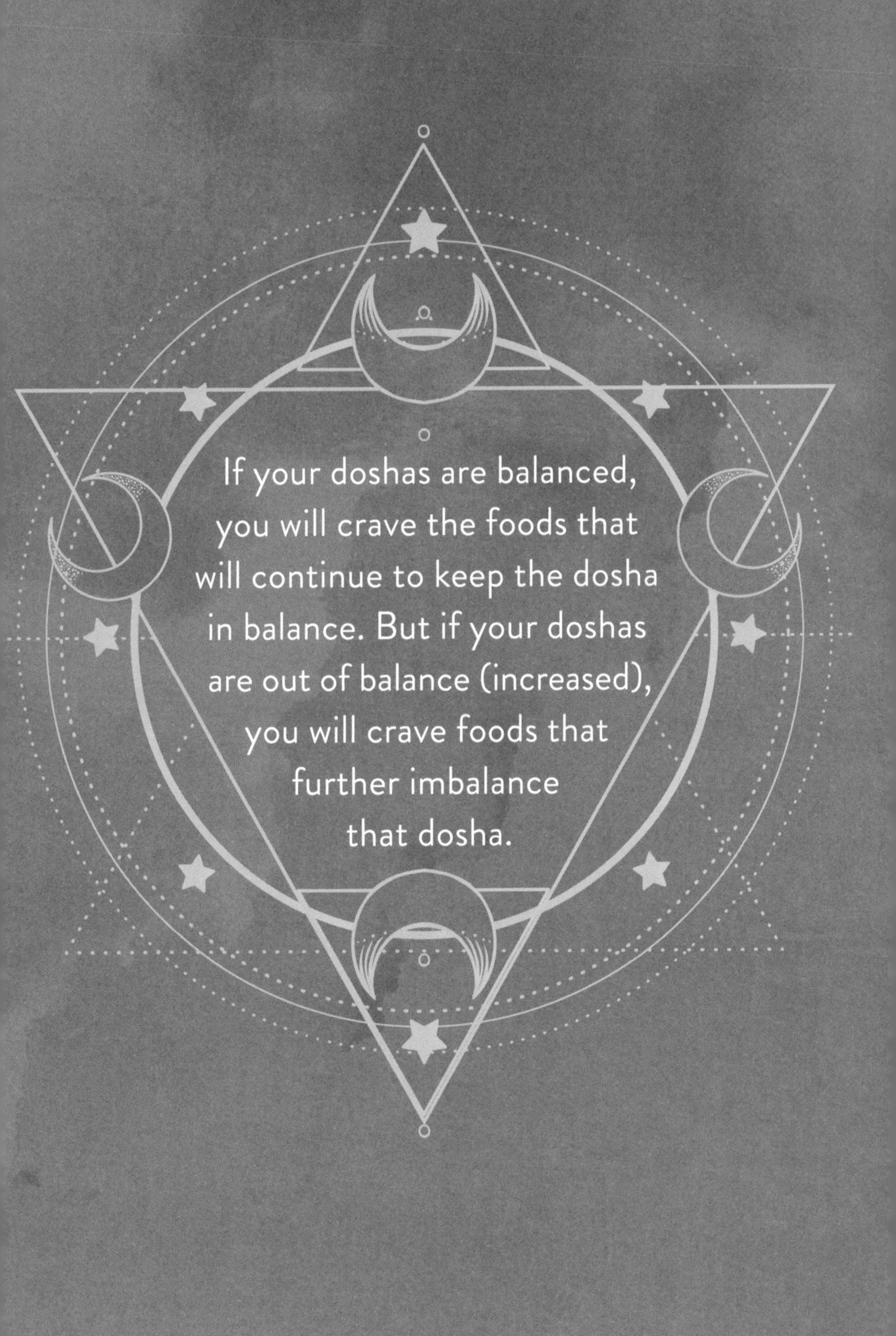

If your doshas are balanced, you will crave the foods that will continue to keep the dosha in balance. But if your doshas are out of balance (increased), you will crave foods that further imbalance that dosha.

Meals for Each Dosha

You knew there were dosha guidelines to eating, right!? Of course you did, because you know that the uniqueness of the doshas matter and everything depends!

Vata meals: Vatas will do best with a consistent schedule for eating three (maybe four) meals a day. Vatas can't eat a lot of food at one time, so they will eat a little bit and feel full pretty quickly. That's fine, but there still needs to be a structure of three meals a day, around the same time each day. The fourth meal could be a small, warm meal of one type of food (like a bowl of rice) around 8:00 or 8:30 p.m. for sounder sleep. Sometimes vatas wake up at night out of hunger and this fourth meal will help keep them sleeping.

What vatas should not do is eat eight to ten snack-meals all day long (vatas love to snack). This only adds to the inconsistency in their digestion and mind-set. Keep a routine of three or four meals a day.

Pitta meals: Pittas need three square meals and they will likely be pretty dang hungry before each one. Pittas have the fire element, so their agni is stronger and more consistent than vatas and kaphas.

Kapha meals: Unless kaphas feel that hunger burn three times a day, they will do best with two meals—and sometimes only one! This is normal for kaphas. That's okay! Rather than letting hunger be their guide, kaphas tend to eat out of emotional or social reasons (because they want to harmonize with the company around them), which can cause them to eat more food than they need. Except, remember, kapha is the dosha that gains weight the easiest. If kaphas eat intuitively, they will discover they actually feel better with less food.

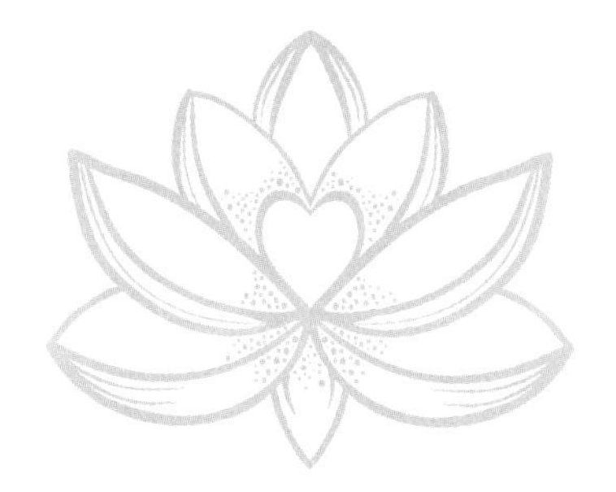

Finding the Right Build

Many people are concerned about weight gain or trying to fix their weight in some way. I'd like to change the word *weight* to *build*—we want to find our right build. Actual weight doesn't always matter, because it's just a number, and I also think "build" is a less judgy way of looking at our beautiful bodies. Essentially, being overweight is having an overbuild of tissues versus optimal build. Due to diet or lifestyle, our tissues can increase beyond our natural size and shape. You know when your body feels good, light, strong, and flexible. You also know when your body feels heavy, sluggish . . . overbuilt! Finding balance in the right build for your unique self is what we are after.

Let's break down the risk of overbuild for the doshas.

VATAS:

Lowest risk of overbuild.

In fact, vatas are likely to become underbuilt, which is why it is recommended they eat foods that are heavy, grounded, and oily, as well as a little bit of meat (when the animal is bigger than the person, it will help build them up!).

Balancing Act: Vatas need foods with the heaviest build and structure because they don't have a lot of structure to start with. If they don't eat heavy "comfort" foods, they will lose steadiness in their mind and their digestion, which is where many vata problems stem from (the colon).

PITTAS: Medium risk of overbuild.	
Because pittas are constantly churning and burning through food, they often feel hungry. They are also highly active, which increases digestive fire further, especially if they are doing intense exercise in bursts, sprints, power moves, or intense competition. In addition, pittas are most likely to eat out of stress. They can use food as a grounding or comfort element. And because they "always feel like eating!" it doesn't feel bad to make that choice—until they find themselves overbuilt.	**Balancing Act:** Pittas, don't abuse your great digestion and overeat. Use your discipline to stay true to a small breakfast, a large lunch, and a small dinner and you'll be fine. Have fruit for a snack if you get hungry between meals. You can reward yourself once in a while with a little piece of dark chocolate. Practice regular meditation or workouts as a solution to de-stress instead of eating.

KAPHAS: Highest risk of overbuild.	
Kaphas have a love affair with food! They love wonderful tastes, the company, the smells, the occasions—they just love it all. Kapha also governs the sense of taste. But remember, here's the rub: Kaphas don't need a lot of food!	**Balancing Act:** The key is to keep portions small, load up the plate with veggies, and skip meals that are too rich, heavy, salty, sweet, or fried.

This dosha breakdown is also why certain diet trends or nutrition plans don't work for everyone—they only work for some of the folks. So, if you've tried various nutrition plans and they don't seem to work for you, that's why! You're not a failure. The foods in that nutrition plan just don't suit you as well as they do someone else. This is why Ayurveda is so customized, because we're all different! Your best guide to find your right build is how you feel in your body.

BRING IT TO LIFE

- Make your own super easy nutrition plan. Make two columns on a piece of paper. On one side list foods that make you feel good. On the other side list foods that make you feel bad. Once you are done, eat the foods in the good column all the time. Omit or really reduce the foods in the bad column. There's your nutrition plan.

- Adjust your schedule to eat at the right time and in the right quantity for a week and write down how your body feels. Keep doing that until you find the right schedule that works for you.

- Practice having a positive mind-set when eating your meals. Leave your stress behind, and just focus on enjoying the food.

CHAPTER 6

Building a Harmonious Mind

The state of your mind is crucial for you to rise, because the mind is what drives us to make right choice followed by right action. Right choice followed by right action is a formula, that if followed consistently, will create optimal health for us. However, if we don't have control over our mind and the direction we want it to go, we probably won't make right choices and actions! The mind will do whatever it wants, and we could go sideways instead of rising. The goal is to create a harmonious mind that leads us to make right decisions and follow through with actions that create our best selves.

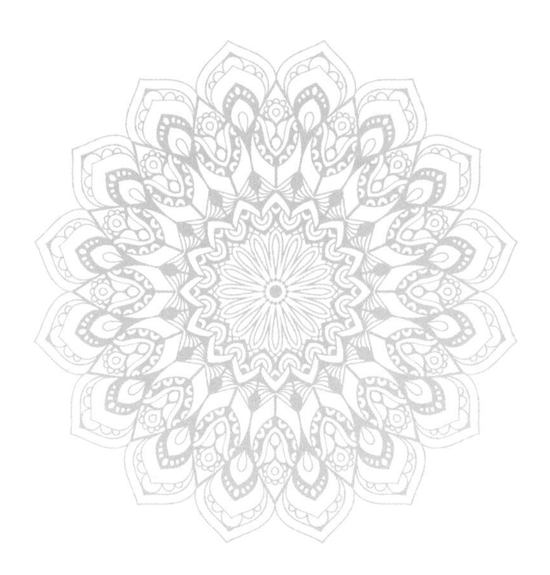

The hardest part for my students isn't learning the doshas or a new routine or food choices—the hardest part is consistently following through with the right actions once they have the knowledge. Follow-through is the thing that trips us up the most because our mind can get in the way. Our intentions are often good (which is the choice), but then we fall apart by not doing the right action (not following through), the things we already know are best for us. This lack of follow-through has nothing to do with the body—it has everything to do with the mind, because the mind tells the body what to do.

When we manage the mind and keep it pure, we make right choices and follow through with right action more often. This purity is the highest quality of the mind and is called *sattva*. When we have a sattvic mind, we seek harmonious solutions in situations, we make the choices that are best for us, we move through our days without harsh words or judgments, and we have more compassion. We could all use a little more sattva, no? Yes. As you rise, in this chapter, you will learn how to create more sattva in your mind.

Because the body is what we can experience with our senses, we tend to put body care first. But the body is just the dressing for the mind and soul.

The body is the vessel. The mind, on the other hand, is the control center, the main driver. The body doesn't do anything unless the mind tells it to. If we don't control the mind, it will drive us all over the place.

You have to be your mind's controller! Don't let your mind go on autopilot! Autopilot is only used as a backup plan. Your life is not a backup plan. Learn to control the mind, and master it. Gain control of the wheel of your mind and *you can do anything*.

A few examples that result from lack of mind control: Impatient, unfocused, scattered, irritated, judgmental, intolerant, anxious, worried, foggy, directionless, bored, restless, undisciplined.

When we control our mind, we become more: Positive, intentional, clear, insightful, focused, disciplined, present, aware, patient, compassionate, confident, sharp, steady, joyful.

The mind pervades the entire body—it's not just in the brain. The mind resides in our heart, our gut, our entire being, and it connects with spirit too. This is how we are a whole being. Mind, body, and spirit are not separate. They work together. When one is out of balance, it affects the other two.

Let's help you manage your mind so you can make right choices and stick to right action.

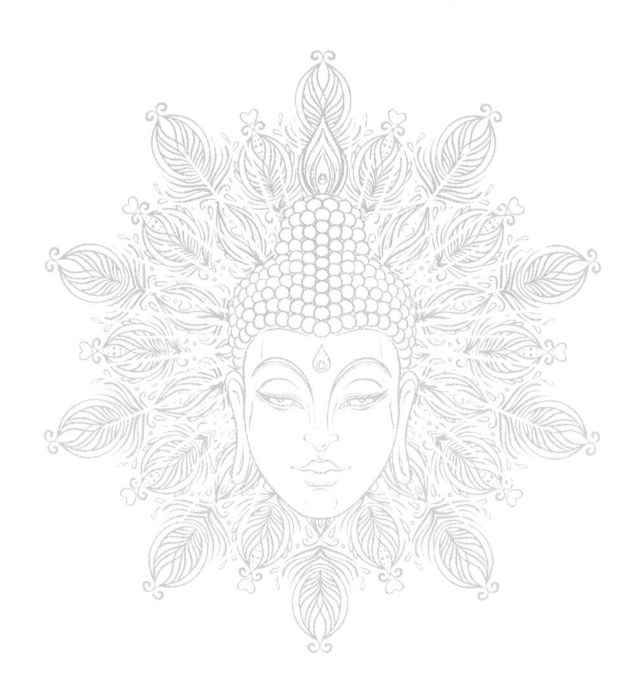

Listen to Your Buddhi

There are several parts of the mind, but the two parts you are most familiar with are the ego and wisdom. Ego and wisdom are constantly sending you messages. Think of ego as the "me, my, I" part of self. The ego is attached to the senses and drives our personal preferences. Ego will tell us what we like to see, hear, taste, smell, and touch. From there, the ego decides whether we like it or not. If the ego does like it, it will call for that thing often, regardless of whether it's good for us; ego just knows it likes it and wants more.

The choices of the ego may or may not be balancing for us. Just because we have a preference toward a certain taste, for example, doesn't mean that the preference is balancing for us.

What we have to do in this case is channel our wisdom, which is our higher self, our soul, our spirit. We call this wise part of our mind *buddhi* (boo-DEE).

Our buddhi is the wise part of the mind that whispers all our right choices to us. Buddhi never steers us wrong. Buddhi is like the angel on our shoulder. Ego is like the kid down the hall in the dorm who just wants to party.

For example, ego-driven cravings might cause us to mindlessly eat a box of Girl Scout cookies. Wisdom says, "Um, you need to stop. You already ate five cookies." Ego says, "But they taste good and I want one more. I can work out extra tomorrow." *munch munch*

Sometimes we can entertain the partier because life should be fun, yummy, and pleasurable. But in order to do our best work and create our best selves, we need discipline! Adhering to wisdom is our discipline. We must stick to our discipline and say, "No, ego. Stop looking at border collie puppies from Australia on social media and write your book."

Learn to check in with your buddhi and do your best to follow through with what it's telling you! Even and especially if you don't "feel like it"; not "feeling like it" is ego. Don't listen to that. In fact, the "I don't feel like it" phrase should be a huge warning flag that if you don't do that thing, you're missing out on an opportunity to create a better you. Buddhi is your higher self and it will never steer you wrong. Ego *can* steer you wrong. Not always, but it can.

The ego is attached to the senses and the pleasure of the senses. If the activity delights the senses, ego is all in (like Disneyland!). If the activity does not delight the senses (like meditation), ego is not interested, and we probably won't follow through. This is why meditation is very hard for some people and falls to the wayside as a practice.

The ego is why most people feel crappy and don't create the life they want! They make autopilot decisions toward satisfying their ego instead of listening to their wisdom. Because right action takes effort and is not always pleasurable, they stay in the ego-pleasure-autopilot mode and don't do what is necessary to evolve. This is where bodies become diseased and our full potential remains stagnant.

Buddhi goes beyond the senses, and if we listen to it, it will help us live better lives. It knows our right choices and cues us to follow through with right action, even if it's not exactly pleasurable.

When we are trying to make big changes, it is essential that we stick to right choices and follow through with right action, even if the actions are not our favorite. Like eating vegetables. Doing a daily workout. Planning our daily three must-dos. Meditating. Practicing breathwork. And being kind or patient, even when we don't feel like it.

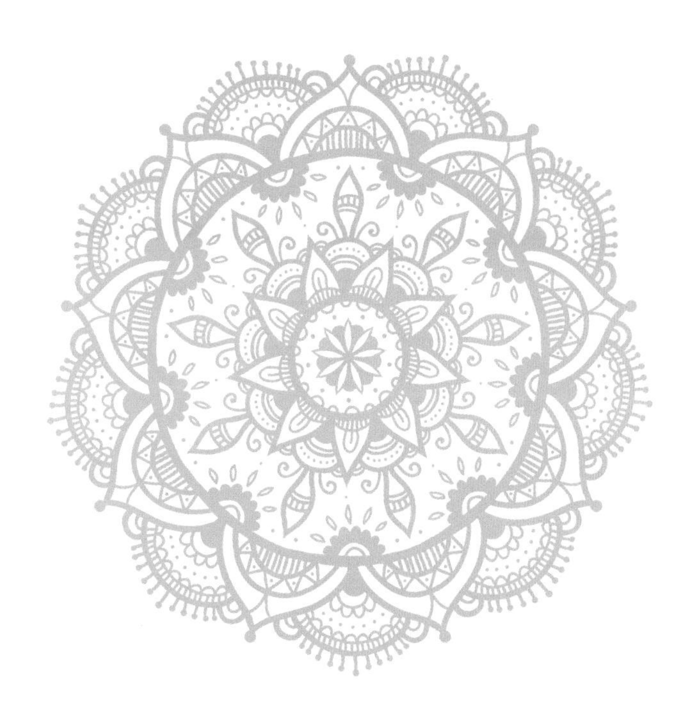

Calm the Mind

There are three huge tools for rising: breathwork, body movement, and meditation. These work to calm your mind. If the *only* things you practice in this entire book are breathwork, body movement, and meditation, you win. This triad of body, breath, and mind is a formula I teach my clients to quickly move out of a negative space of worry or stress—and it works every time.

I'm so passionate about these three things (breathwork, movement, and meditation) because they pulled me out of burnout when I saw no other way out. I had an overwhelming schedule and lifestyle with limited time, but I created a few minutes in the morning for these things and everything improved. If you are struggling with burnout or overwhelm, start with one of the following practices, daily.

USE YOUR BREATH

The fastest way to change the mind is to use the breath because the nostrils are the quickest passageway to the brain. We can calm the mind almost instantly by breathing deeply, slowly, and intentionally.

Think about this: if we don't breathe, we die real quick. We are used to taking the breath for granted because *it keeps us alive without us having to actually do anything*! Hang on, can we give a quick shout-out to our breath? "Thank you, breath, for keeping me alive!" If you utilize the breath as the main tool for mind control, your body, your mind-set, and your days will completely change, my friend.

If you find yourself in a moody space feeling negative, worried, cloudy, or a little down, use your breath. It will help in a pinch! You will feel better as soon as you use your breath in a conscious way again, because of the direct passageway from the nostrils to the brain!

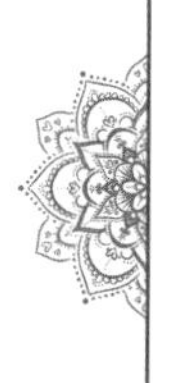

BALANCING ACT: *Try using your breath now to calm your mind. Sit up straight, feet flat on the floor, mouth closed. Take ten deep, slow breaths from the lower belly. Go ahead, I'll wait. See? That required no equipment and took maybe two minutes. Welcome to the power of your breath. How do you feel?*

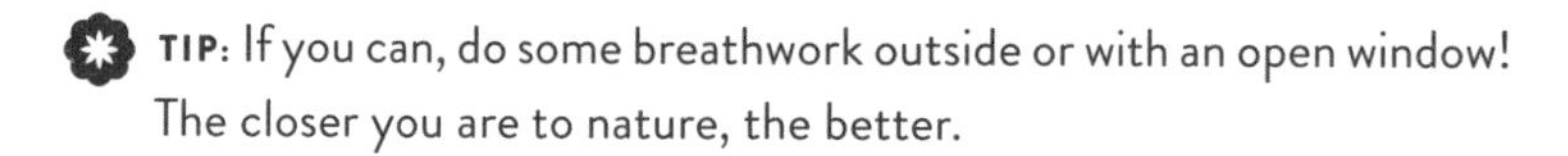

TIP: If you can, do some breathwork outside or with an open window! The closer you are to nature, the better.

MOVE YOUR BODY

The second fastest way to change the mind is to move the body. Mind, body, and spirit all work together, so if you influence one of the three, you will influence the other two. Therefore, using the body directly affects the mind and lifts the spirit.

When we move our bodies, we enliven the tissues and boost circulation, and heat increases. When heat increases, so does agni (that's a good thing!) and we sweat. A little sweat is good because sweat is one of the three waste products (poop, pee, sweat) and expelling waste products each day is necessary for good health and a happy mind.

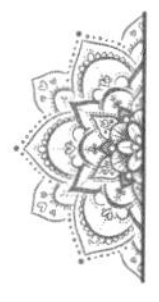

BALANCING ACT: *Move your body. Stand up and do ten squats or thirty seconds of jumping jacks. Then clap your hands five times when you're done.*

MEDITATION

Once you've done both breathwork and moved your body, your mind will be ready for meditation. Meditation is one of the best ways to calm your mind. It will be easy. You can just sit for five to twenty minutes and breathe. Meditation takes discipline. Remember, meditation is void of the senses, which makes it hard at first because there is no "sensation." The reward comes after the practice, and you might have to do it for a while to feel the benefit.

This is why it's so hard for people to actually stick to a meditation practice because it feels like . . . nothing. Ego doesn't like nothing. Ego likes sensation and action.

But here's exactly why you need to do it. Because life is full of sensations and action. That's why, as a counterbalance, meditation is essential to gain mind control.

Practicing meditation as a consistent discipline will train your mind to keep doing other hard things. And we need that because in order to evolve, we need to do the hard things in life.

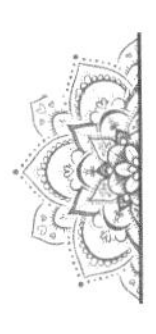

BALANCING ACT: *Practice meditation daily, even if you start with five minutes.*

Practicing meditation as a consistent discipline will train your mind to keep doing other hard things.

Feeding Your Senses

Ayurveda uses our five senses (hear, see, touch, taste, and smell) to receive information from the outside world. What we do with our senses gets digested by our body and our mind. A simple example is when we see something gorgeous or inspiring and it makes our mind feel better. We have digested that experience that came from our sense of sight and it is now in our memory.

However, we also digest seeing something violent, sad, or disturbing. We might even say, "I can't unsee that!" because what we see can deeply affect our perceptions and thoughts. Depending on the emotional impact, the mind replays events as if they were really happening, again and again. If it's negative and scary stuff, that's what our mind will be fed and that's what our emotions, perceptions, thoughts, and beliefs will be made from.

Think of the senses as mind food. The senses drive how we perceive everything, including our inner, outer, and physical world. Just like with food, we need to feed our senses high-quality sensory input in the right quantity. If you over-, under-, or misuse your senses, your mind and body will become imbalanced.

Remember, walk the middle path.

PRACTICES TO CARE FOR THE SENSES

If you've never thought about using your senses as a powerful vehicle for healing and balance before, hooray! Now you know. You have an amazing opportunity to consciously feed your senses positive ingredients, every single day. What you feed your senses creates your perception of reality. Here are some ideas on how to nourish and balance yourself through the senses.

See/Eyes: Limit screen time and turn off any screen at least sixty minutes before bed. Too much screen time engages and agitates the mind.

Hear/Ears: Listen to pleasing sounds, like music that makes you feel good, positive words, motivating and inspiring stories, or the sound of your child's voice. Stay away from too much stressful news or talk radio, depressing music, or gossip sessions at work.

Touch/Skin: Give hugs and snuggles often to people you love, apply warm coconut oil to your skin, pet your dog, or enjoy a warm shower or bath. Stay away from water that is way too hot or way too cold, and never hug or touch someone you don't like.

Taste/Tongue: Savor every bite of food and chew well. Avoid eating too fast, eating too much, or canceling out an entire food group. Enjoy a balance of tastes in your food, including sweet, sour, salty, pungent, bitter, and astringent.

Smell/Nose: Enjoy pleasing, natural smells from the outdoors, turn on a diffuser with essential oils, or bake cookies to share with your neighbors. Stay away from smoke, exhaust, pollution, and chemical smells as found in some household cleaners.

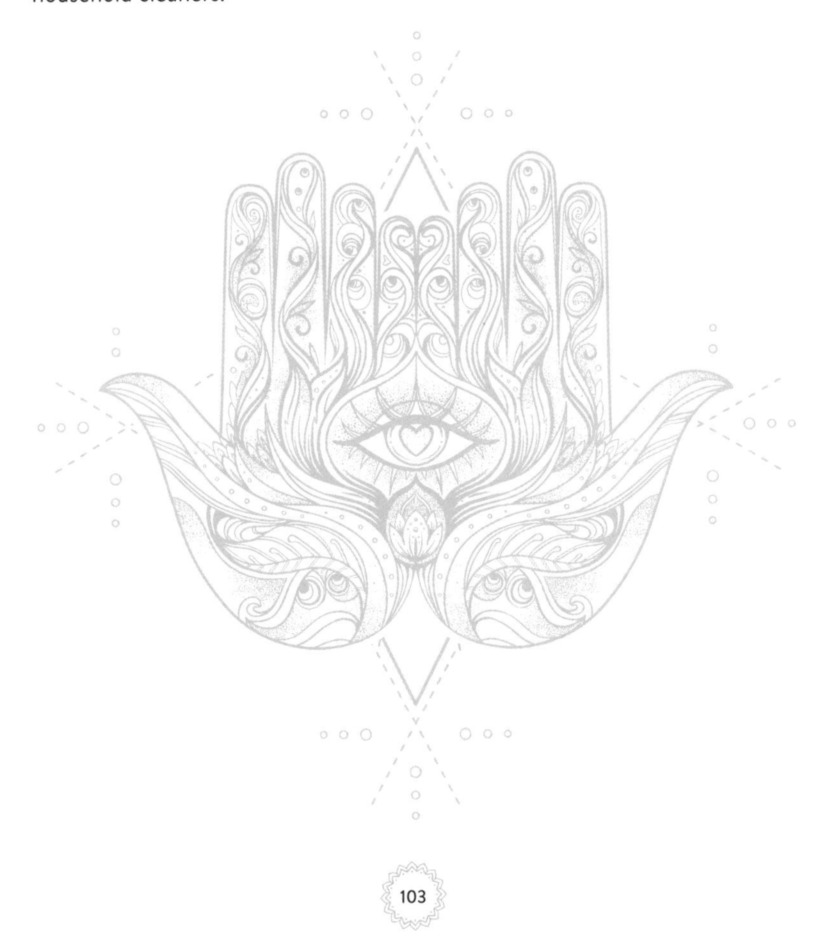

DETACHING FROM THE SENSES

Now that you know how to care for your senses, I'll throw you for a loop, because we have to learn how to master and detach from them. Our power comes in when we have mastery over our senses and go beyond that experience. It's the inner knowing that no matter what we see, hear, taste, touch, or smell right in front of us, there is much more going on under and above the surface!

Unlike the body, the mind is capable of detaching from the senses and going into the unknown, like dreams, thoughts, beliefs, and realms that are not tangible.

Think about all these cool things that happen that you can't capture with your senses: How about conception! Tulips suddenly poking up out of snow. The ocean floor. Your gut instinct. Aging. A wound healing. Hair growing. When someone thinks of you at the same time you think of them. The time it takes to learn something. A changed attitude.

Gosh, we could come up with so many things. My friend, go beyond the senses. There are intangible forces at work at all times. Trust what you cannot experience with your senses. Trust that it will be okay. Trust that the universe is working in your favor and that will calm your mind.

As your mind rises up to create your full bloom, understand that there is so much more beyond the five elements and the doshas. Your true essence goes far beyond the physical—and your mind is the driver to take you to that higher potential.

BRING IT TO LIFE

- What do you see, hear, touch, taste, or smell that takes you down a wrong path?
- When can you tell yourself to have trust beyond the senses?
- What choices in your life feel like ego is overriding buddhi? What is your buddhi (wisdom) trying to get you to do (same messages over and over) but you refuse to listen and make the change?
- Whatever your answer is here, it is gold! Where you refuse to listen and change is exactly where you need to go. Override your ego, follow your wisdom instead, and you will make major progress. You are rising!

Part 3

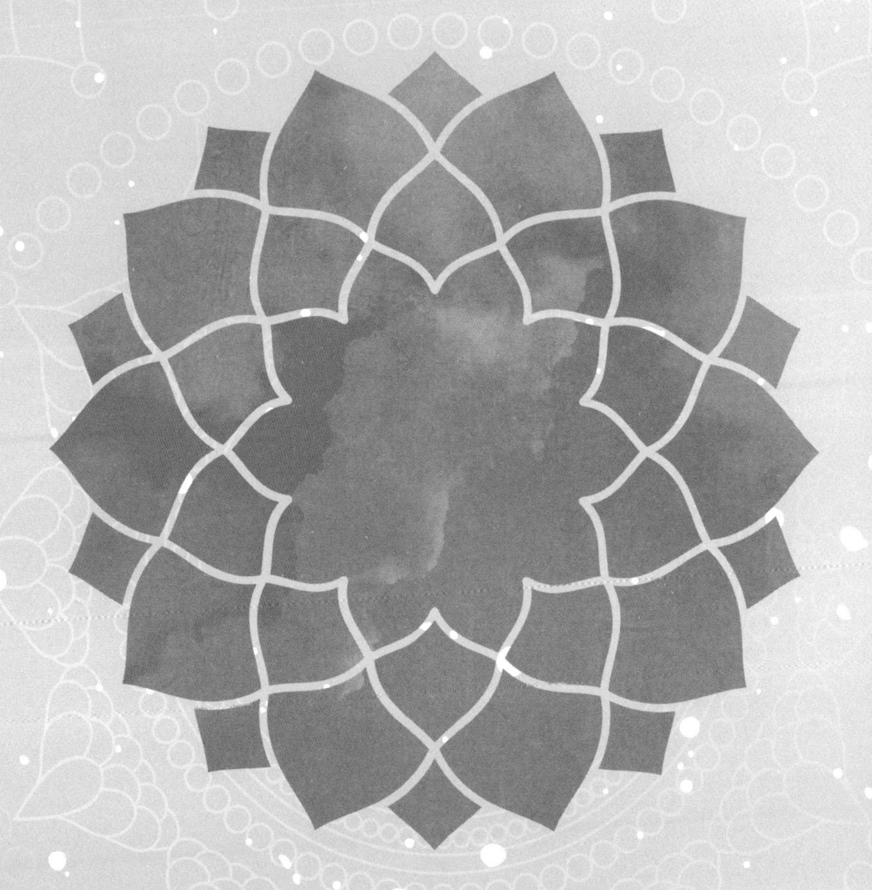

BLOOM

CHAPTER 7

How You Will Screw Up

(AND OVERCOME IT)

Yay! Here you are with strong roots and you've gathered new practices to help you rise, too! You're ready to bloom, my friend! The blooms will keep you flourishing by giving you daily energy-enhancing tips and reminders to keep you in your flow and help avoid potential pitfalls and screw-ups.

Now that you have discovered all this wisdom and new practices, you are probably full of gusto and promise to make positive changes for yourself. Woohoo! But here's a wee bit of truth. Despite your best efforts and desires, you will mess up. You will have some setbacks or things won't go according to plan—that's just how life is, right? Don't beat yourself up about it. Instead, anticipate the potential pitfalls, so you can identify them when they pop up and rebalance with your improved mind-set and new habits.

Self-Negotiation

There's a strong chance you'll read this book, love it, and then negotiate yourself right out of doing any of the practices! It will go kind of like this: "I know I should work out this morning, but it's cold out and I could just fit it in later this afternoon or after work. Or maybe I can just skip today and do it tomorrow . . . " *raise your hand if you have ever had thoughts like this* Totally, we all have!

Allow me to be your coach for a second. Anytime you've heard yourself say, "I know I should but . . . ," that is you negotiating yourself out of something that will be awesome for you. Don't get stuck in that trap!

Let's be real. If you were stoked to make changes, you would already be doing them. Your new habits won't be super easy at first (although some will be!). But that's okay. With a little discipline, you will be able to do the difficult things for the sake of creating the health and life you want.

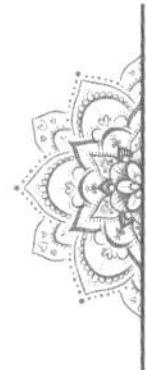

BALANCING ACT: *Act fast. Leave little to no space between the decision and the action, because in that space, you will come up with excuses. And then you're doomed. Negotiating creates time and space between you and the choice, which makes it easy to weasel out of something that's difficult (discipline) or you don't want to do (procrastination).*

The key to any of these potential screw-ups is to catch them before or while they are happening so you can turn them around. This is not always easy and takes full awareness—this is the mind control we talked about in chapter 6. No autopilot. Take control of your mind and create a new outcome. The more you do this, the better you'll get, and eventually the balancing acts become your defaults instead of the potential pitfalls.

Negative Talk Tracks

That little voice living inside your head isn't always positive, is it? That little whisper of doubt or critique says, "I'm just not good enough," or "I'm such a hot mess," or "You suck at that, so don't bother trying." These negative talk tracks can totally screw you up, bring you down, and stifle right choices and right action.

Your job is to master the negative talk track (master your mind!) and turn it into a neutral or positive message. Negative talk tracks are just mental patterns you recite over and over based on experience and/or beliefs. The truth is, you're bigger, better, and stronger than that sassy talk track, so work bit by bit to master it.

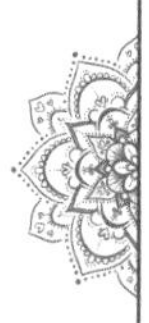

BALANCING ACT: *When you catch your mind going down a negative path, tell yourself "new choice!" Then, come up with new choices until you get to something that serves you. Let's use writing a book as an example.*

A negative thought:	**New choice!**	**New choice!**
"There's no way I can write a book in such a short time frame."	A stressful thought: "I can probably pull it off if I stay up until midnight every day until it's done." This is a stress thought and while it's slightly better, it still doesn't serve me.	"Dude, I write all the time. I can do hard things. I'm a creator. I was born to do this, and I have enough time if I buckle down and focus. Keep going!"

TIP: "New choice" also works to stop yourself from negotiating! If you start making excuses to avoid doing healthy practices, say "new choice!" and begin again.

Putting Other People's Agendas Before Yours

It's not a bad thing to be helpful; in fact, the reason why we're all here is to help each other and be of service. But when you are at the beginning of creating a healthier, new life for yourself with new practices, you need to focus on yourself and practice for a while before it becomes your foundation.

It's easy to slip into the pattern of saying yes to everyone and everything and filling the space you fought so hard to create for yourself with their stuff. Help them, sure. But only if you have the time and energy after you have done *your* practices. Don't fill your time with their agendas or your life will be their agendas.

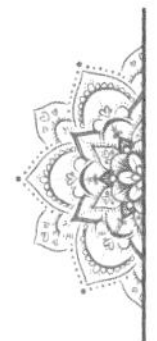

BALANCING ACT: *Hold the time and space for your practices as sacred. If you are susceptible to letting other people run all over your schedule, self-care, time, agenda, to-dos, and must-dos, then this is for you. *raise hands**

Here are a couple of ways to tactfully navigate saying no.	**The quick no:** Immediately say, "Oh thanks, but I can't make it." Done. Do not let yourself ponder. Nip it in the bud. It doesn't mean you are a bad person; you are choosing how you want to spend your time and your life. That is powerful and rooted in truth!	**The slower no:** If you are uncomfortable with a quick yes or no, then say, "I'd love to help with the school rummage sale, but before I commit, let me check my calendar first. I'll get back to you tomorrow." Feel the difference in the decision. Make a choice. And get back to that person tomorrow so it doesn't linger.

Don't slog in a wishy-washy space because that's going to create a loose tie for you and may weigh on your energy. Just give it a "Heck, yes!" or a "Thanks, but no," quickly, so you don't have to worry about it anymore. Be decisive (looking at you, vata). And preserve time to get your things done without giving away all your time and energy to others while leaving yourself last (looking at you, kapha).

You have the power
to make a new choice
at any time.

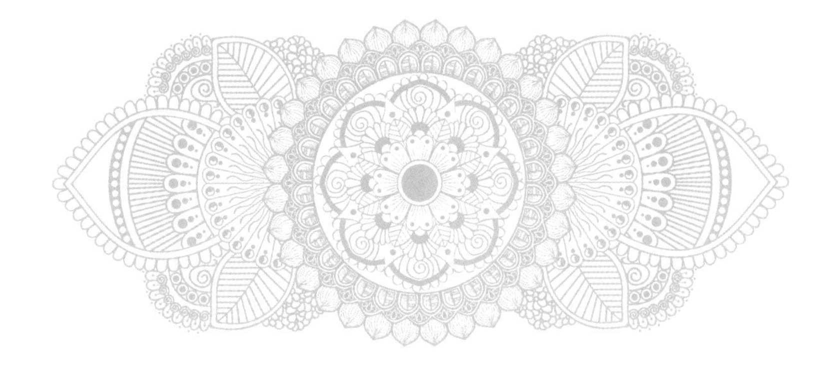

Overcommitting to Your Practices

I get it. You are motivated and want to make fast and awesome changes because you are a high achiever who can tackle difficult things. So true, you *are* and you *can*! But please do not commit to a big list of practices and try to work on all of them at one time. If you try to change a lot of things at once, you'll fail to stick to them. And when you fail to stick to them, first of all, you'll feel bad about yourself and second, it will be harder to get the gusto to start again.

Your confidence will tank (vata), or you'll beat yourself up (pitta), or you'll just stop altogether (kapha). We need to make changes slowly and one by one.

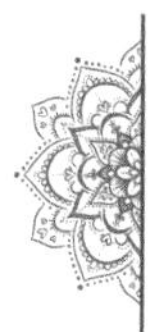

BALANCING ACT: *Do not commit to doing any more than three practices (max!) at any given time. In fact, I recommend doing one or maybe two. Vatas, do just one and crush it. Let's set you up for success.*

Expectations

Oh yes, our expectations can mess us up big-time. How many times have you been disappointed or twisted up about something you thought would, could, or should happen, but didn't? *everybody's hands are up* If you think back to real disappointments (go ahead, think. Maybe make a list of the big ones in the last year), you might discover that the disappointment was not about the thing that happened but about your expectation of the outcome. You are disappointed you didn't get the raise (you expected at least a little something). Your mom can't babysit today (but she's never busy on Tuesdays!). The client didn't go with your proposal (you expected you were the clear choice). Only two students came to your yoga class (you expected at least fifteen). Your partner didn't take out the trash (you expected them to because it's Thursday). There's a backup on this street again (why is there always traffic on this street? Keyword is "always"; change your expectations).

It's one thing when someone promises or commits to us and then lets us down—that's a legit expectation letdown right there. But it's completely different if we, in our dreamy, maybe perfect-scenario minds, really hope or expect a certain outcome. This just causes disappointment *and* can actually reduce any feelings of winning. Because not every situation is a losing one—there are great things that happen in each scenario, even if it didn't go the way we wanted or expected it to.

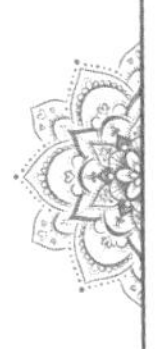

BALANCING ACT: *Embrace a learning mind-set. When you enter a situation, be ready to learn from it. The outcome doesn't matter as much as what you can take away from it. Too much traffic at that stoplight? Maybe there's a better route. No better route? Change your expectations so your mind stays at peace. This stoplight will always have a backup, so accept it and crank up some good tunes.*

BRING IT TO LIFE

- What do you already negotiate yourself out of, repeatedly? *(Note: If you just changed one of these habits and stuck to it, you'd have a new life. Your wisdom is telling you, repeatedly, that this is what you need to do.)*
- What might you need to prepare ahead of time so you don't have time for negotiating? Example: Setting out your workout clothes in a pile the night before so all you have to do is grab them and put them on.
- What are your most common negative talk tracks?
- Use "new choice" (as many times as it takes!) to get a neutral or positive statement instead. *(Note: These should be rooted in truth and not based on made-up scenarios.)*
- Is there any one person or situation that consistently steals your time? If so, how can you say no or put their agenda in a time/space that works better for you?
- What consistently disappoints you? Write it down. Change your expectation because that thing will likely happen again and again unless you have a direct influence over it. How can you accept it or learn from it?

CHAPTER 8

Life-Enhancing Boosters

As you go through your Ayurvedic journey, I thought you could use some life-enhancing boosters whenever you get stuck, need a quick remedy, or have to reboot. I've made it a practice in my busy lifestyle to sneak in frequent yet short practices to reset my mind, body, and spirit, often! Whether it's five minutes of breathwork, a ten-minute walk up a super steep hill, a visualization, or even just closing your eyes to get clear on what you need to do next, these mini boosters will revive you and keep your energy high so you can accomplish what you need to.

The fastest ways to change
the mind is to use the breath
and move the body.

Breathwork: 10-5-10

1. Set a timer, if you choose, for 5 to 10 minutes.
2. Sit with your back straight, feet flat on the floor.
3. Close your mouth and breathe through your nose.
4. Inhale for a count of ten, then hold for a count of five.
5. Exhale for a count of ten, then hold for a count of five.
6. Repeat for 5 to 10 minutes.

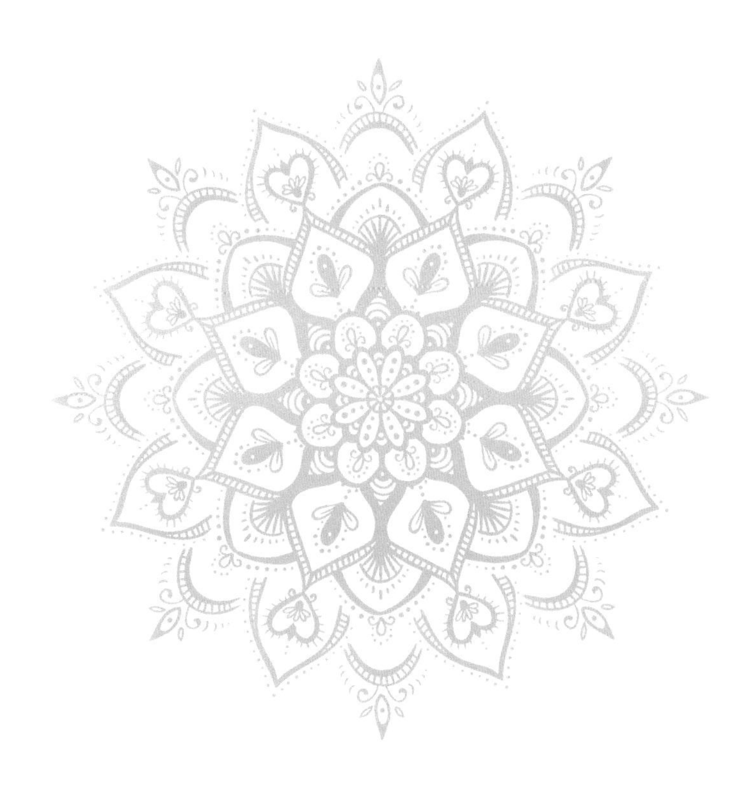

Meditation: Have a Seat

1. Set a timer for 5 to 10 minutes. Make sure it's a pleasant "wake up" sound, like gentle bells, chimes, or harp music.
2. Sit with your back straight, feet flat on the floor. Or lie flat on your back (no pillow), arms next to you, palms up.
3. Take ten deep and slow inhales and exhales, breathing from your lower belly, not your chest.
4. Let your breath return to normal and observe the ins and outs . . . until the timer goes off.

If this is hard for you—good! It means you are changing. Don't judge, just practice. You might feel squirrely at first, but allow yourself to practice a few times, without judgment or expectations, and you will start to crave the stillness. Be gentle with yourself. This is your time to sink in. Make it a daily practice, though, because you'll benefit and change a little more each day. Our bodies need this stillness.

TIP: There are some great apps for guided meditations that you can search online. You could also make a playlist with nature sounds or gentle yoga-esque music and let it play while you close your eyes and breathe.

Take a Moment of Transition

We are busy people, playing several roles in one day, from parent to boss to spouse. As we go through the day, we may drift between these roles seamlessly, but sometimes we drag the residual gunk along with us from one role into the next. For example, we may go from a stressful meeting at the end of the day and bring it home to our family and snap at our kids for no reason. Or maybe we have a difficult conversation with our teenager right before we are supposed to present at a board meeting.

We need to get good at ending one role, to transition completely fresh into a new one so that we can be of good service for the people who need us next! If we take a conscious moment, we can create a transition to separate ourselves between these various roles, so that we arrive in each moment fresh and fully present, leaving any residual gunk in the past. It doesn't take a lot of work or time; it just takes mindfulness. Just five to ten seconds makes all the difference.

1. Choose a role you play daily and make a conscious choice to arrive in that role completely clean of any other energy that has affected you that day.
2. Then, choose some short words as the person you want to show up as in your new role. That's it!

TIP: You can use visual cues to help you, like when you sit in a certain chair, you transition. Or when you close the car door, you transition. Or maybe just a pause in the bathroom mirror in between meetings. Maybe you have a sticky note on your laptop as a reminder. Or go digital and use your calendar reminder as a signal that it's time to move from one role to the next.

Cut the Cords

As we show up to serve each day, we interact with many different people and our energy can get tied to their struggles, stresses, emotional baggage, and whatever they are carrying around with them. Not many people use transitions to enter a situation with full presence, so there's a high likelihood you may be on the receiving end of somebody else's vibrational soup! That's not good because you'll end up feeling like you have to take on or fix their problems.

Your energy can get tied to theirs in what I like to visualize as strings or cords. All the strings and cords come out from you and attach to them, which you may not want! Whether good ties, stressful ties, needy ties, whatever, you need to detach from them to keep your energy pure so that you can serve and feel your best.

1. Visualize all the energetic cords attached from you going outward to all the people who need you or whom you've engaged with recently.
2. Then visualize cutting them all. You can visualize giant invisible scissors or the cords dissolving or just completely releasing the cords. Be creative! This is your cord-cutting ceremony.
3. When you are cut free, take three big inhales and exhales to fill yourself with your own energy from head to toe. Woo! You're free!

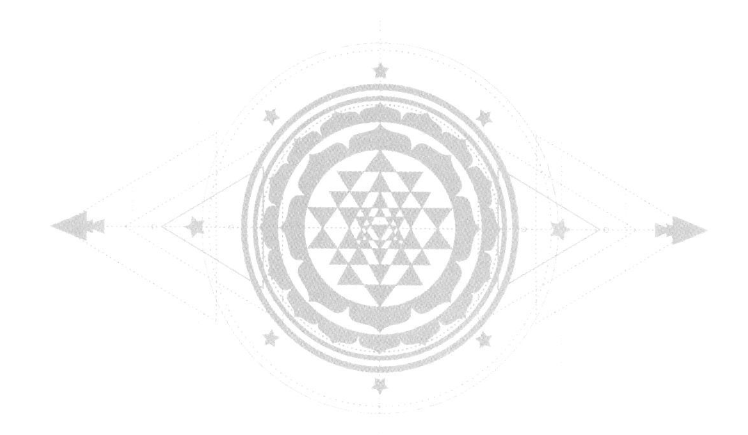

Protection Shield

When somebody comes to you uninvited and just vents, complains, and throws all their emotional garbage at you, you can leave the situation feeling spun out, depleted, even violated. I call this an "energetic hangover." It's these moments when we get caught off guard (with certain people we may be able to see it coming) by someone else's bad attitude, crabbiness, or traumas. Protect yourself with an invisible shield so their junk doesn't get to you. I learned this technique in a meditation class.

1. Visualize that you have a protection shield. In meditation class, we use a giant rose to hold in front of us. Make it your own safety shield and choose whatever gives you power. My shield is a dome, the color of rose quartz, and it drops down from the sky over my head and covers my body, like a big pod. I can see through it.
2. As this person talks to you, listen to their words with full presence, but let their words and energy bounce off the shield or fall in front of you, so their negativity does not enter your space.
3. Ah . . . now you can listen fully, but without absorbing any of their negativity.
4. Energetic hangover averted!

Grounding Cord

If you ever feel like your mind or energy is zipping fast like a kite without a string, or you have a self-doubt in a moment where you need to be confident, use your grounding cord to give you a sense of security.

1. Sit straight with both feet flat on the floor, back straight.
2. Visualize a cord coming down from the base of your spine. Again, make it your own. This cord could be a chain or a thick rope, something strong that will hold you very secure.
3. Close your eyes and visualize the cord coming from the base of your spine, going all the way down through the ground, and reaching the center of the earth. The cord holds you secure and grounded to Mother Earth. You are secure, you are safe, you got this. You are exactly where you are supposed to be right now. Tell yourself these words as you feel yourself heavy and grounded.
4. Take ten slow, deep breaths and then open your eyes.

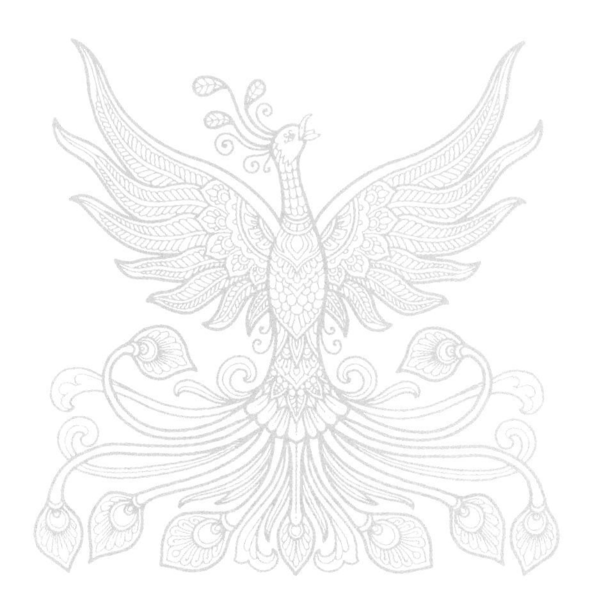

Move Your Body

Get your daily exercise on! If that's hard for you, stick with me, because I'll make it doable and enjoyable. We don't want very intense exercise daily because that could deplete the tissues. We also don't want anything too easy because it won't make an impact.

In Ayurveda, there is a right and wrong way to exercise. The right way to exercise is to work at an intensity enough to create sweat on your brow and in your pits. Start with fifteen minutes if you need to and work up to thirty minutes. That's it. In the Western world, we tend to obsess about exercise by either exercising too much, which causes stress on the tissues and puts our agni into overdrive, or not exercising nearly enough. These are extremes. We want to walk the middle path, even with exercise. Just enough to create a sweat is all you need to get the benefits.

The rules for everyone: Do some kind of exercise daily for at least fifteen to thirty minutes that creates a little bit of sweat. For instance, my without-fail daily exercise is a twenty-to twenty-five-minute hilly run with my dog. I don't even think about it, I just do it. However, it's important to note that the doshas have different requirements for exercise.

EXERCISES FOR VATA

VATA	
Vatas will want to:	Jump, run, bounce, and be speedy. But this increases their already light and lively, fast nature, which is not balancing for them. Vatas don't have good endurance, so they will start with a quick burst and fizzle out quickly if they don't pace themselves.
Vatas need to:	Keep both feet on the ground, use slow and intentional movements, and use their own body weight or light weights for strength building. They also tend toward dryness, which can make them tight or inflexible.
Best exercises for vatas are:	Yoga, barre classes, hill walking, lifting light weights, low-impact cardio, martial arts, stretching, meditation (see what I did there? Sit still, vatas).
Potential pitfalls:	Vatas have a hard time keeping a consistent exercise routine. Just do the same thing at the same time of day, every day, until you are bored out of your skull. Then you can bring in something new.

EXERCISES FOR PITTA

PITTA	
Pittas will want to:	Do high-intensity, super sweaty, competitive, challenging exercise. If it doesn't make them hurt or sweat, they will think it's not worth their time. However, pittas are already strivers in so many other areas of life that doing high-intensity exercise as a habit will keep their mind amped up, when they really need to calm it, cool it, and soothe it.
Pittas need to:	Use exercise for enjoyment and stress relief, not more competition. They should avoid any exercise that will overheat them and avoid exercising during pitta time, which is from 10 a.m. to 2 p.m.
Best exercises for pittas are:	Yoga, barre classes, hill walking, lifting light weights, low-impact cardio, martial arts, biking, swimming, and just-for-fun group sports.
Potential pitfalls:	Pittas are the most motivated and committed to exercise (unless their work gets in the way), but they will have a hard time not overly kicking their own tushy. Anything too hot or competitive will increase those qualities in their mind and body.

TIP: Pittas have sensitive skin, so bring your own towel to the gym or workout class because if you wipe their bleachy white towels on your face, you could get red-faced rashy irritations. It's happened to me and I thought something was wrong with me. Just bring your own towel.

EXERCISES FOR KAPHA

KAPHA	
Kaphas will want to:	Be a spectator and clap. But it's not what's best for them.
Kaphas need to:	Move their body vigorously, daily. It doesn't have to be long; it could be fifteen minutes, as long as it's fun and full of lots of movement. It's crucial to get them to sweat—they are made of so much water and they need to lose some of it to maintain their balance.
Best exercises for kaphas are:	Cardio, dance class, spin class, power walking, hill walking, or anything that is fun, sweaty, and highly active. They do best with a bubbly accountability partner to inspire them to do it daily.
Potential pitfalls:	Exercise is the very hardest thing for kaphas. They just don't like to move and will want to talk themselves out of it, but it's really necessary. They will feel light on their feet and like a million bucks when it's over. They need tight accountability to make exercise a habit, so working with a trainer or a group class can help. Or kaphas can just crank the music at home and have a dance party in their room for fifteen minutes—just sing along, boogie, and call it good! They will feel amazing. So that their mind doesn't get in the way, kaphas can create a bookmark folder of three to five online exercise links so they can always find them easily and quickly when they are ready to work out.

Take the time to reset
your mind, body, and spirit.

BRING IT TO LIFE

- What is one area where you need to transition from one role to the next? Maybe it's at the end of the day on your commute home, where you shed the "work" role you play so you can open the door at home, happy to see the people you love there.
- When are moments when you need to use your protection shield?
- What is the best time of day for you to cut the cords?
- When do you feel you need to use a grounding cord?
- Add these to your journal pages so you can use them as tools every day!

CHAPTER 9

Keep Bloomin'!

So here you've gone all the way from the roots, you've worked hard to rise, and you're up to the tippy top of your beautiful blooms. Great job! You have probably had to adjust your schedule or maybe your food intake; perhaps you had to have a mind-set reset or just bring awareness to the things you are doing. Maybe by now you are truly listening to your body and what it's calling for. 'Atta way! Your journey is unique to you and you're already making fantastic progress!

In any case, this journey of balance, good health, and building a life on your terms is a long one. It's never finished. Many of us think of working on our health as a finish line. Kind of like, "Once I fix this problem, I'll be good." But it's more like, "Once I fix this problem, I'll be so grateful, so I'll keep doing the things that prevent it from coming back."

Good health is a lifelong practice. We need to work on it a little bit each day, like the dishes. If you don't do the dishes, you end up with a sink full of dirty plates, and then you have to tackle that smelly mess as you say to yourself, "Why didn't I just do this when it was a manageable size?" Yes. That is just like your life.

Let's keep you blooming in your mind, body, and spirit. There are three major things to live by to keep yourself blooming.

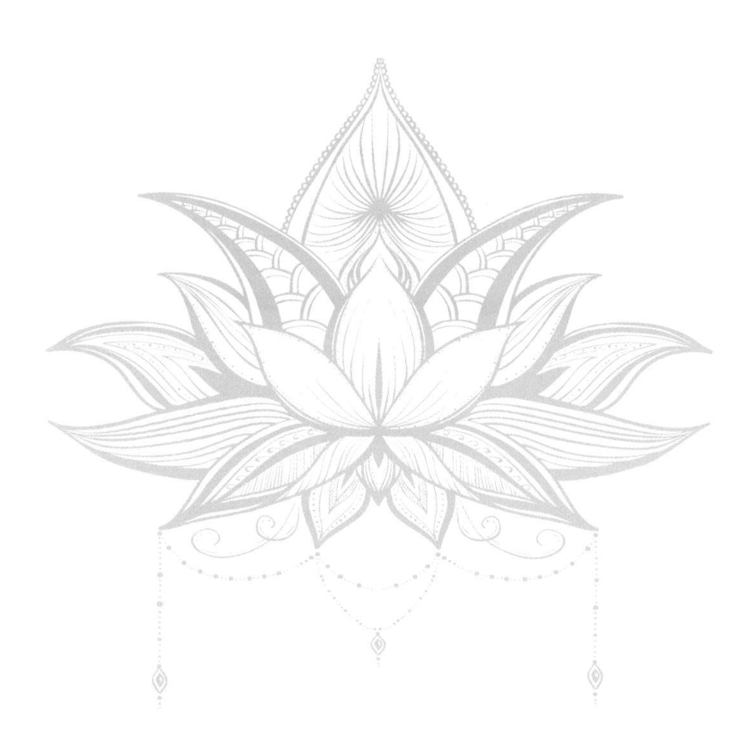

Health is not a finish line.
It's a lifelong, daily practice.

Live a Life Filled with Prana

Prana is our vital life force. *Vital. Life. Force.* Understand the power of those words. When prana is lacking, I see it in people's postures, their gait, their dull skin, their tired and zoned-out eyes, their strained smiles—they are exhausted and lifeless. Without sufficient prana, we will feel, look, think, and act lifeless! Take this life-sucker seriously and pay attention to this one.

If we lack a strong vital life force, how are we supposed to show up for others as our best self as a parent, boss, partner, child, friend, and all the roles we play in life? We can't. It is essential that we are conscious of what we put into our bodies, because the more prana we take in, the more alive we will feel.

Fill yourself with prana! Prana is the reason we are alive, and prana is the thing that will keep us feeling that way. Prana is our breath; it is oxygen. Take time to breathe consciously every single day. Prana is in foods from nature, so choose to create a diet filled with seasonal foods that grow in your area. Prana is in water, so choose water more than you choose sugary or caffeinated drinks. Prana comes from the sun, so take a break and get outside instead of sitting under office lighting all day. Prana comes from the rain, so don't complain about the rain—thank it.

Take Care of Our Mother Earth

Remember, the planet and us are made of space, air, fire, water, and earth (macrocosm and microcosm). The state of the planet determines the state of us. The more purity in the earth, the more purity in us, because 100 percent of what surrounds us and what we consume comes from our planet.

We don't get another option, so we need to take care of Mother Earth. She keeps us alive. If she is poisoned, we will be poisoned. If she is depleted, we will be too. If she is on fire, we will burn. If she floods, we will wash away.

She's bigger than us, and we are at the mercy of her great powers, but I would also argue that she is at the mercy of ours. Put it at the front of your consciousness because in order to keep you healthy, you must help keep her healthy. Our great Mother Earth provides *all* of our life force. Without a well-functioning mother (earth, or even you), the rest cannot survive.

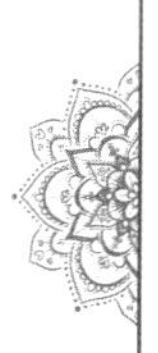

BALANCING ACT: *There are countless ways to protect Mother Earth. Choose something that is simple, daily, and doable for you. Get produce from the local farmers' market, if you can. Grow some fruits or vegetables and share them with neighbors. Reuse rainwater. Plant trees. Volunteer for environmental cleanup days. Bring reusable bags to the store. Drink water from the tap. Compost. Insert thousands more ideas here. Whatever you choose, a little action goes a long way. Let her be your caretaker and take care of her too. And be sure to thank her, every single day.*

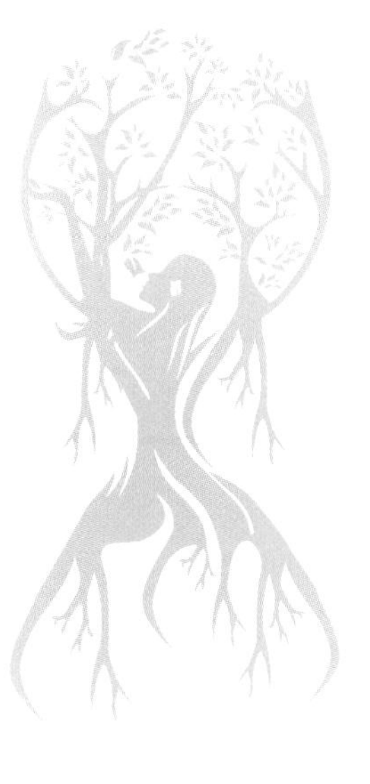

Put Yourself First!

Do you feel like you put yourself last on your to-do list? Well, the last thing on the list is usually the least important. And you don't belong there! Who's the most important person in your life? Everybody at one time should shout "me!" Yes, that's right—*you*! Because when you are full up on energy, eat good food, have a balanced schedule, and move your body daily, hot dang, you're an unstoppable force! You'll be a force of love and grace if you learn to take care of you first! It's not selfish; it's so you can serve others. We are here to be of service, and we cannot be of service if we are falling apart. We will fall apart if we keep putting ourselves last on the list.

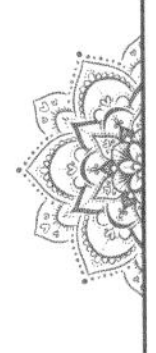

BALANCING ACT: *Use the mantra "Me first!" The phone, social media, news, or email does not come first. Before you do anything else, put your self-care first (twenty minutes of exercise, breathwork, meditation) and get it done in the morning, preferably during vata time, or at least before anybody else in your house wakes up. If you live alone, you are primed for this. If you have little kids, this is harder. Try to get up before they do (that's what I do). If that's not possible, then recite the "Me first!" mantra in your head so that you don't forget to do your self-care at some point in the day. If you want my guidance through this, see the link for my Bloomin' Balance System on page 143.*

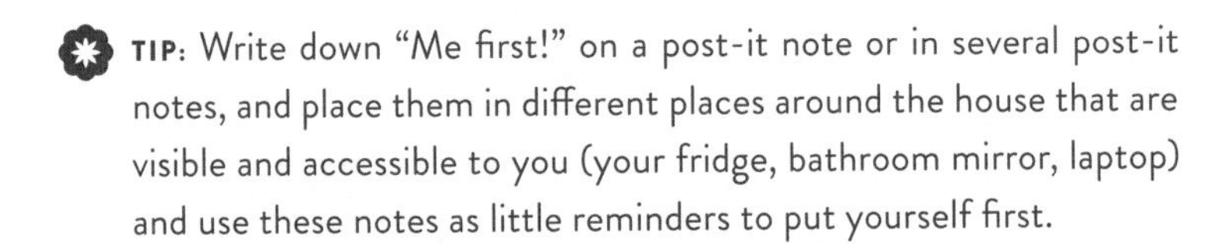

TIP: Write down "Me first!" on a post-it note or in several post-it notes, and place them in different places around the house that are visible and accessible to you (your fridge, bathroom mirror, laptop) and use these notes as little reminders to put yourself first.

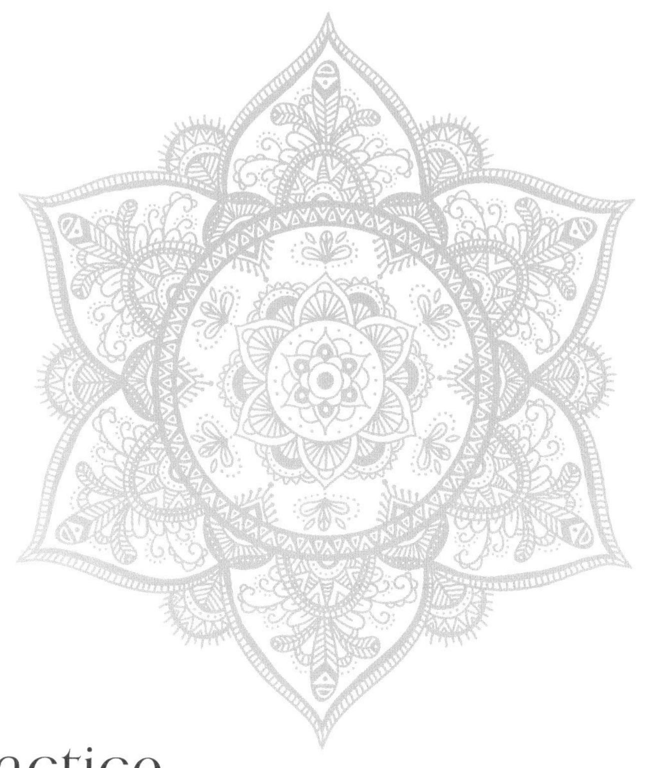

Practice

Mindfulness is our whole life! It's not just sitting on a yoga mat for ten minutes a day and hoping for the best. Our life is a walking, breathing, living meditation that is to be learned from and evolving every single day.

You must begin to practice. This book is full of practices, but reading about them will not change your life. What you read will fuel you with knowledge and hopefully inspire you to take action.

Right now, choose one or two practices from this book that you can get started on immediately. Find a time slot in your schedule and commit to them. Commit to making them a habit. Go back and flip through the chapters right now to find a balancing act and just choose one. Knock it out of the park with consistency and commitment. When you get good at that one, add another.

Don't know where to start? Then I suggest you start with this combo: breathwork, move your body, and meditation (see chapter 8) and get it all done in one chunk.

Now, I know that life can get in the way of your practice. If you can see the obstacle ahead, you can plan to get around it before it impacts you.

Take a big *inhale*. Good. *Exhale*. Good. Hey, you did it! You worked your way through a whole Ayurveda book, and it made sense to you! You can do this! You have all the power you need to change your life! Well, except for the things you can't change.

There are many superpowered things we can do that we haven't done before. There are many ways we can influence our own health and lives and the community around us. Except for the things we can't change or influence. There might be parts of you that drive you nuts. Perhaps it's your hair, your skin, your thighs, your nose, your *fill in the blank.*

The highest quality of the mind is called *sattva*. Sattva is purity. It seeks to create harmony, and it is the quality that helps us adhere to right choice and right action. Sattva accepts what is. When we can accept ourselves (and others, situations, things that don't go our way) exactly as we are, there's a wave of peace that comes with it. It is what it is. If we cannot change it, we can accept it. It is one of the most calming things we can do for our mind.

Acceptance is one of the best ways we can honor ourselves and celebrate who we are as a unique, never-again-replicated, divine arrangement.

Let's take a moment to accept and give thanks to all parts of ourselves, including the parts that we wish were different. "Thank you, body! Thank you, mind! Thank you, soul!" Let us stop wishing things were different, masking it, or distorting reality. Let's stop trying to make our bodies something they are not. Let's accept our beautiful bodies and love them for giving our souls a place to reside. Remember how significant you are, just as you are. You are already enough.

If you just got a little teary, that means your heart chakra opened up. We touched on something big and it just changed you. You'll never be the same. Woohoo! Here's to evolution and creating a life on your terms!

My friend, you're ready. Get going. Well done and big hugs all around!

RIGHT NOW, PUT YOUR HAND ON YOUR HEART AND RECITE OUR BLOOMIN' VOW

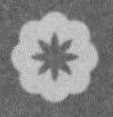

From this day forward, before I do anything else,

I WILL TAKE CARE OF ME.

I deserve it. I work hard.

I AM ENOUGH *just as I am.*

I love me!

Every day I will take at least fifteen minutes

to MOVE MY BODY.

I will CONSCIOUSLY BREATHE *for ten minutes.*

I will DRINK ENOUGH WATER.

I will CALM MY MIND WITH MEDITATION *for ten minutes.*

I will choose to EAT THE BEST FOODS *I can find.*

I will GIVE MYSELF TEN MINUTES *before bed*

TO REFLECT *on the day and* GIVE THANKS.

I will do these things daily so I can serve.

It is essential that I take care of me.

I LOVE ME.

THANK YOU FOR ME.

Author's Note

Thank you for reading this book! Thank you to all my readers, students, and supporters! So many of you have stuck with me for over a decade and I cannot say enough about what you mean to me. Every day I say a prayer of gratitude and I zing it out to all of you. Thank you to the newbies who are learning Ayurveda for the first time and being here with me; be sure to share this with anyone who needs it. If you want to know more and get deeper into Ayurveda, check out my other book, *In Your Elements*, on Amazon or check out some of the book extras on page 143.

This is just the beginning, my friend. Put on your rainbow mind-set while walking on the middle path as you keep bringing Ayurveda to life.

Visit my website at *heymonicab.com* for online classes and subscribe to my podcast, *Bringing Ayurveda to Life.*

Connect with me on the socials @HeyMonicaB:

- Youtube Channel
- Instagram
- Facebook

Love,
Monica B.

Acknowledgments

Major kudos and thanks to my editor Keyla Pizarro-Hernández, publisher Rage Kindelsperger, creative director Laura Drew, and the rest of the Quarto crew for creating this book with me! Endless thanks and humble gratitude to my great teachers, colleagues, and all the people who have helped me in my life. I want to be fully inclusive and if I make a list, I will miss some, so I'd rather send out a big, magical, star-filled thank-you to all. Even people who showed up for a blip in time have been life-altering and I am equally as thankful for them as for the people who have helped me for years and years. So, for all the people who have loved me and supported me for decades, as well as you helpful angels who showed up out of nowhere, as a blip, I send my eternal gratitude.

My heart is full, pink, and fuzzy with bursts of glitter for my beloved family. Tres and Alella, thank you for loving me through all my wild ideas, agendas, and deadlines, and for giving me wings to share my soul and service. Mom and Don, thank you for always telling me to go for it. Auntie Jam, thank you for your endless hooty laughs about funny life things. Go-Mom, thank you for a lifetime of your loving care and silly fun. And to the rest of my family who are far in miles but close at heart, love to all.

Book Extras

Let's continue the conversation! This book is just the beginning of our time together. Remember, life is long! We have to stick together and keep helping each other reach our highest graces as we use our roots to rise and create our blooms in this lifetime!

Find the daily routine, breathwork videos, dosha cheat sheets, sattva cheat sheet, quote printables, and more at *www.heymonicab.com/ayurvedaforlife/bookextras.*

For a step-by-step guide on a twenty-minute life-changing routine, check out my Bloomin' Balance System, a busy person's guide to daily balance (move your body, breathwork, meditation) at *https://www.heymonicab.com/bloomin-balance-system.*

If you want to know your dosha(s), take my quiz at *www.heymonicab.com/blog/dosha-test.*

About the Author

Monica Bloom has been enthusiastically sharing Ayurveda since 2008, but it was only after living at the intersection of a stressful corporate job, a 3-hour daily commute, new motherhood, and a side hustle, that Monica became the expert at tucking Ayurveda neatly into a busy modern life. That craziness resulted in the ultimate burnout, so she used her Ayurvedic know-how to renew her health, create peace in her mind, and exude joy each day. And then she started leading others to do the same.

Because of her journey, her sweet spot is teaching busy go-getters how to enrich their mind, body, and spirit so they can have fun achieving their goals, create their best health, and love their life! Monica's purist delivery of Ayurveda's ancient wisdom fused with practicality and humor makes Ayurveda accessible and fun. Monica firmly believes when Ayurveda is made simple, you have all the power to transform your life.

Monica also authored the book *In Your Elements*, and as a corporate coach, brings wellness into the workplace for Fortune 100 companies. She lives in the California sunshine with her husband Tres, daughter Alella, and brown dog Rio. To learn more, visit her website heymonicab.com and follow her Instagram @heymonicab.